Praise for
The Cancer Book

*"For those of us who have been in the 'cancer club'—
as survivors or family members—the stories in this book are not just
brilliant and moving and often funny. They reach down in a variety of
ways and touch us in the deepest place, where fear and hope reside."*

~Jonathan Alter, Newsweek

"Chicken Soup for the Soul: The Cancer Book *conveys an impressive
spectrum of cancer stories and poems written by patients, spouses,
children and caregivers."*

~Cynthia Nixon, actor and cancer survivor

*"After I heard those dreaded words, 'You have cancer,'
I found that the stories of fellow survivors offered me and my family
much needed hope. This book serves as a wonderful resource
to those coping with this disease."*

~Doug Ulman, three-time cancer survivor and
President/CEO, Lance Armstrong Foundation

Chicken Soup for the Soul

for the **Soul**.

The Cancer Book

Chicken Soup for the Soul: The Cancer Book; 101 Stories of Courage, Support & Love
by Jack Canfield, Mark Victor Hansen, David Tabatsky

Published by Chicken Soup for the Soul Publishing, LLC   www.chickensoup.com

Front cover photo courtesy of iStockPhoto.com/Graffizone.

Cover and Interior Design & Layout by Pneuma Books, LLC
For more info on Pneuma Books, visit www.pneumabooks.com

Distributed to the booktrade by Simon & Schuster. SAN: 200-2442

Publisher's Cataloging-in-Publication Data
(Prepared by The Donohue Group)

Publisher's Cataloging-In-Publication Data
(Prepared by The Donohue Group, Inc.)

Chicken soup for the soul : the cancer book : 101 stories of courage, support & love / [compiled by] Jack Canfield, Mark Victor Hansen [and] David Tabatsky. It's just a word / by Elizabeth Bayer.

    p. ; cm.

With: It's just a word / Elizabeth Bayer.
ISBN-13: 978-1-935096-30-6
ISBN-10: 1-935096-30-3

1. Cancer--Patients--Literary collections. 2. Cancer--Patients--Anecdotes. I. Canfield, Jack, 1944- II. Hansen, Mark Victor. III. Tabatsky, David. IV. Bayer, Elizabeth. It's just a word. V. Title: Cancer book

PN6071.C25 C45 2009
810.8/02/0362196994   2008944059

PRINTED IN THE UNITED STATES OF AMERICA
on acid∞free paper
16 15 14 13 12 11 10   03 04 05 06 07 08

Chicken Soup for the Soul

for the Soul®

The Cancer Book

101 Stories of Courage, Support & Love

Jack Canfield
Mark Victor Hansen
David Tabatsky

CSS

Chicken Soup for the Soul Publishing, LLC
Cos Cob, CT

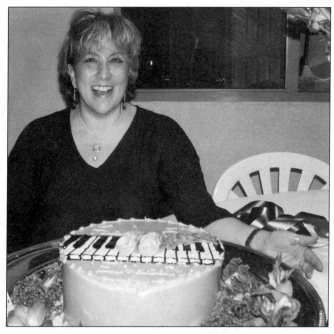
www.chickensoup.com

Contents

~For Better and For Worse~

~Unfinished Business~

~Dreams and Nightmares~

~Partners~

~Loss~

❽

~Fear and Hope~

❾

~Letting Go~

~Into the Light~

Foreword

To the world you may be one person,
but to one person you may be the world.
~Anonymous

I almost wish this book didn't exist. If nobody had cancer in the first place, the world would be a better place. But the disease rages on in all its incarnations and we deal with it head on.

And deal with it, we do. This book is a testament to that.

101 stories of courage, support, and love is an understatement. Each and every author reveals a unique piece of the human spirit—from finding strength they never knew they had to feeling an absolute fear of losing control; from discovering what true support and love means to realizing they are all alone; from finding faith to losing it and finding it again. In all of these stories, for better and for worse, we discover that everyone, male and female, young and old, rich and poor, has a story to tell about cancer.

Many of these essays are uplifting while others may not be easy to digest. But all are authentic and honest, and they reflect the staggering reality of the cancer world.

When I was first asked to compile this book, I thought it should contain a cross section of contributors: patients of all ages and backgrounds, their loved ones and friends, doctors and nurses and research technicians, those who have reached good conclusions and those who, unfortunately, have not.

The daunting task of reading all of the submissions became almost unbearable. I found myself absorbing the authors' struggles and grew exhausted trying to make sense of it all. But eventually, I became energized by the stories, inspired by these remarkable testimonies. I discovered that cancer affects each of us differently and our reactions are often surprising.

Melissa Sorensen, of Woodbridge, Virginia, wrote of her husband, "When you're diagnosed with cancer four times, it is not uncommon for family, friends, and coworkers to share their utter disbelief. I saw shock on people's faces when Scott would say, "I'm trying out a few different cancers in hopes of finding one I really like."

Dorian Solot, of Albany, New York, grew used to people staring at her bald head, but one day, when asked by a stranger in a hushed, I-feel-so-sorry-for-you tone, "Did you lose your hair?" she smiled and replied, "Lose my hair? Oh, no. It's just invisible." The stranger stared at her in shock. Then, she started to giggle, and so did Dorian, who wished her a good day and headed out the door.

Bonnie Davidson, of Marion, Massachusetts, struggling with the consequences of her cancer, overheard her daughter telling her boyfriend, "My mom has no breasts, no uterus, and no hair, and my dad still loves her. That's the kind of love I want."

That's the kind of love I have discovered throughout this book. Now it's your turn.

~David Tabatsky

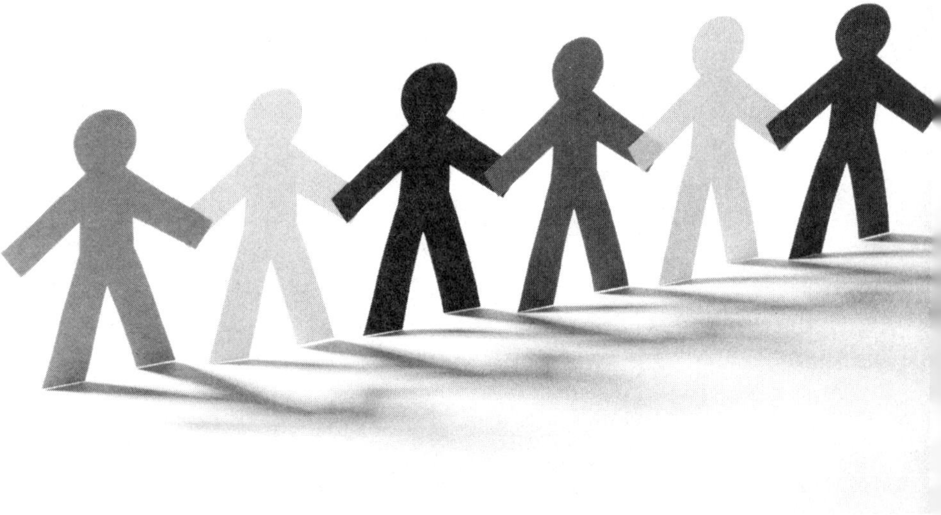

The Cancer Book

Out of the Blue

Yesterday is history. Tomorrow is a mystery.
Today is a gift.
That's why we call it the present.

~Babatunde Olatunji

Chicken Soup for the Soul

Booger

Out of the blue, I discovered something in my nose. It was bleeding. I went to the doctor. She sent me to the hospital. I filled out the papers and got in line. I stayed overnight. They took a biopsy. I threw up all night. Next morning, they sent me home.

Two weeks later, I went back for the diagnosis and to discuss what form of treatment I would have.

One doctor said, "radiation."

"Hmm," I replied.

"On the right side of your face all the nerves will die and your right eye will drop and your neck will turn blue," he continued.

"Oh really?" I responded.

I decided I needed a second opinion.

The next doctor said, "I think reconstruction is the way to go."

"What's that?" I asked.

"We remove your nose and then we remove the cancer," she began, without blinking an eye. "We pull away the right side of your face, just above the eyelid, over to the left side of your face and the left side then goes back over the right and then we can reconstruct your nose."

"No kidding?" I said. "And you've done this before?"

"All the time," she replied.

I decided I needed a third opinion.

The next doctor told me that I would need chemotherapy for twenty minutes a day, five days a week, for six weeks. Knowing myself pretty well after sixty-four years, I'm pretty sure I can't do anything on time, five days a week for six weeks straight.

"Well, if you do nothing, you'll die," he said, quite matter of factly.

"I have a loving wife and great kids," I began to say out loud.

"That's nice," he replied.

"Is there an alternative?" I asked.

"No," he said, so firmly that I almost believed him.

"What about laser treatment?" I asked, showing off my research skills.

"There is no difference between radiation and laser," he replied.

"Oh really? What if you slice down the side of my nose and go in and cut the booger out?"

"Booger?" he asked, not understanding my choice of words.

"Yeah, the booger, the piece in my nose. The cancer!" I answered, remembering that I was living in Germany and not everyone knew what a booger was.

He said, "I'll call the surgeon. If you sign a paper to the effect that if he finds any complications we will reconstruct your...."

"Wait a minute," I interrupted. "With all due respect for you and your treatment plan, I'd rather drink muddy water and sleep in a hollow log."

With that remark, I got up and left the interrogation room. As I passed through the lobby, I saw all these folks waiting for their turn with the men in white coats. At this point in my life, I have learned there are three things bad for you: white sugar, white bread, and men in white coats.

While walking home, I realized I had no choice but to develop some form of self-healing. I needed even more information on my type of disease. Since I'd been meditating for many years I totally believed in the magic of the world around and within us, so I prayed for guidance.

It became very clear that for a nose operation I needed to be in a hospital in the country, away from the city. I was gonna need fresh air. Luckily, in Germany one has a choice of places to go, so I called my dentist, who lives in a little village in the center of a part of Germany I can't pronounce, and I told him about my problem.

"Bob, I'm a dentist," was his first response.

"Yeah, I know, but I need help," I replied. "I need some alternative thing."

"We just have a small hospital here," he continued.

"I know, but I like the vibe," I said.

"Okay, come down," he answered. "I'll set you up with the professor."

At the hospital, the professor doctor sat me in this kind of electric looking chair and he looked in my nose and he looked some more and finally he said, "Do you want me to do this?"

I said, "Yes, that's why I'm here."

"Are you sure? Because I could do this."

"Yes, I'm sure."

"Then, why did you call a dentist?" he asked. "A dentist can't do this but I can."

"I called him because he's my friend," I replied.

"I know," the professor doctor said. "He can't do it, but I can."

"Right," I said.

I figured anyone that crazy is either great or really crazy.

A couple of days later, I had the operation. The professor doctor came to my room to check my nose. I looked like Karl Malden on a bad day, but I couldn't see a mark, a scar, nothing. Before I was ready to go home to Berlin he came back in my room, very excited.

"I got it all!" he cried.

"How did ya do it doc?" I asked.

"Forget it," he said. "You'll never understand."

Two years later, I found out. He had done it by hand. While I was in dreamland, he'd reached up my nose and done his magic. For five hours he worked. He put a piece of tendon in my nose to cover the hole from the removal of the tumor. In short, he took an entirely different direction than any of the other doctors were ready to take.

He did what I wish all doctors would do: he made a choice based purely on my health and not on what was best for the insurance and pharmaceutical companies.

I had prayed for magic. I had changed my diet. I had chosen the belief that we're all going to die so I worked on that spirit before I saw the crazy professor doctor. And now, with great pleasure, I still have a nose from which to happily remove a booger.

~Bob Lenox

The Brave Spider

"But I'm only twenty-five years old."

"I know."

"I've got two boys to raise by myself."

I sat in Dr. Anderson's office, trying to convince him that I didn't have time for cancer, that I couldn't work it into my schedule and that I simply would not be told that I had it.

"I'm in my twenties, for God's sake," I shouted. "No one my age gets cancer."

Dr. Anderson stood quietly by while I cursed, cried and yelled, and when I didn't have it in me anymore, I collapsed onto his sofa, wishing it was just a bad dream. My mind was racing with the finality of it all.

"Jamie, are you okay?"

Dr. Anderson's voice was smooth and calm. I resented him immediately.

"Am I okay?" I screeched. "No, I'm not. What am I going to do?

What was I going to tell Aaron and Ryan, my boys, my buddies, my little babies?

"This is not the end," Dr. Anderson said. I could hear a touch of panic in his voice as he saw the blood draining from my face. "We can talk about surgery and medication. You're young; you can get through this."

It was as if I was hearing him from inside a tunnel. My mind latched onto key words like, "not the end," "surgery," and "get through this."

"What do you mean?"

"We can do a partial mastectomy."

Dr. Anderson spoke quickly to hold my attention.

"You're a large-breasted girl so this type of surgery may do you well in the long run but the main thing is, we can get the cancer."

His eyes were soft and I knew he meant what he was saying. I looked down at my chest as I breathed and saw that he was right. I was a large-breasted woman. I can see my legs. Now they're gone. There they are again. Now they're gone. I was at least a DD with enough to spare.

"When?" was all I asked.

"As soon as possible," he replied. "The less time we give it to spread the better, and judging from your mammogram, we stand a good chance of getting it all."

"So," I hesitated, "there is a chance that you might not."

"There is always that chance, yes," Dr. Anderson said.

A week later, I went under the knife. After surgery, Dr. Anderson explained that he thought they had gotten it all and I would now be a small C cup in breast size. I spent the next several days relearning to walk because the change in my chest size had thrown my balance off.

I arrived home to find my sons, Aaron, who was nine years old, and Ryan, who had just turned four, waiting at the front door with flowers and homemade cards. They led me to the bedroom, helped me into bed and then crawled in with me. Aaron read me a story while Ryan huddled close. We fell asleep together.

I had made it through surgery, but the hard part was just beginning. I started chemo three days later. Each time, I spent several hours in my bathroom afterwards, vomiting. Being sick to my stomach was hard enough, but I also had more than fifty stitches around my breasts. The chemo made me tired and sick and it didn't take long before I began to regret the surgery.

"What do you mean, you wish you hadn't started this?" my

mother demanded. "The alternative is death; is that what you want for your boys?"

"Maybe," I shot back. "Maybe they'd be better off without me. Look at me. I have two jobs, I'm going to college, and we're living with roommates to make house payments. I'm a mess, and I'm tired. Maybe they'd be better off with their father."

"You don't mean that," my mother said quietly.

"No," I said. "I don't."

I watched Aaron and Ryan out the window, playing with a bug. Ryan was trying to pick it up and Aaron was systematically slapping his hand away. Ryan adored a good bug.

I didn't want the boys to live with their father but I was reaching my limit.

Seven weeks later, I came home from chemo one day and headed straight for the bathroom to throw up. An hour later, I slid to the floor and felt like I would stay there, wedged between the toilet and the shower, and cry myself to death. The boys were out so I could wail as loudly as I needed and no one would be the wiser. I tried to stand up but couldn't find the strength. I managed to grab a bottle of painkillers the doctor had prescribed with about twenty left. I popped the cap and poured them all into my hand.

"You can do it," said the voice in my head. "You can end all the pain right here."

As I lifted my hand, pills and all, to my mouth, I heard the front door open. The boys were home. I put my head down on the toilet seat and cried. My hand began to sweat on the pills. Ryan appeared in the doorway, a smile on his face and his hand held out proudly. When he realized I was crying, his smile disappeared and he began to cry too.

He ran inside the room and threw his free hand around my neck. He wasn't about to let go of whatever he had in the other hand.

"Ryan, Mommy is okay. I was just sad for a minute." He sniffled and tried to read my face, to see if I was telling the truth. I did my best to smile. Ryan smiled too, and hugged me.

"It's okay, Mommy," he cooed, rubbing my hair.

I asked him what was in his hand. He burst into a grin, and as he held it out I screamed in surprise. In Ryan's small hand lay a Daddy Longlegs, which he displayed proudly. At first I thought the spider was dead but then it moved.

"Ryan," I said sternly. "Take that thing back outside." He looked up at me suddenly concerned.

"But Mommy," he protested. "He's special, look."

I looked. It was a spider. I wasn't getting it.

"I named him Harry. He only has five legs, see." I looked at Ryan's new pet and sure enough, he only had five legs.

"Harry might have run into a monster spider or a bird and it tore off his leg," Ryan explained. "But Harry keeps on living with just five legs. Look Mommy, Harry doesn't give up."

I sat there in awe. I suddenly realized how selfish I had been to even consider giving up. Here was my baby boy looking at the world with such innocent eyes and learning some very big lessons from a bug, of all things. I hugged Ryan close for a long time. He hugged me back just as hard and for just as long. As we sat there holding each other, marveling over Harry, the five-legged spider, I dropped that handful of pills into the toilet and flushed it. My younger son was saving my life.

~Jamie Farris

It's Not the Answer.
It's the Question.

As the doctor pointed at the blue, shape-shifting blobs moving across a darkened screen, I tried to be analytical even as I was feeling devastated. I tried to appear hopeful, while all I heard was one word: malignant. Ever since my doctor had said the c-word along with my name, both in the same sentence, all I really saw was my life slipping away, vanishing before my eyes.

My thoughts raced in a hundred directions. I'm only forty-four, too young to leave behind the people who love me. And my five Labradors, my Jack Russell — what about them? Would they feel as if I'd abandoned them? Wonder what they'd done wrong?

For the past year, I'd been dealing with my mother's battle against her own inoperable cancer. Then, a week before my surgery, my father was rushed to the hospital for an emergency procedure, a complication from his colon cancer.

I'd blinked, and suddenly we were all struggling for our lives.

I wondered: Why me? A ridiculous question when you think about it, really, because there's no logical answer. Cancer is what happens to other people, people who don't take good care of themselves, people exposed to insidious carcinogens or deadly asbestos, people living under power lines. People just like me.

I heard voices. Not the kind that come from an unbalanced

mind—just the opposite, because these voices came with clarity, and that was the problem. The truth had never been an issue for me. I'm a curious person. I've often been criticized for trying to make sense of the senseless. But this cancer coming out of nowhere, I realized, would be my toughest test of all.

I tried to accept the challenge but didn't get far. If there was a lesson, I just wasn't learning it. If there was a blessing, I didn't feel it. There was no inspiration, no revelation. No matter how hard I tried to make things fit, I couldn't. At the end of the day, I still had cancer and no suitable explanation.

Was I going crazy? Had the stress from my diagnosis forced some sort of break with reality? It seemed possible. On the outside, my world was in turmoil. It would have been easy to fall apart, but instead, I did the opposite. I pulled everything together.

Facing my own mortality forced me to prioritize.

I heard something, nothing audible, but it was very clear and very powerful, and there was no mistaking the message: Cancer wasn't just about me; it actually involved everyone else. My world began shifting toward a more universal consciousness. In life, there are no bad experiences, only lessons. It's easy to get caught up in a crisis, but if you're only watching the ball, then you're missing the game. Shifting your focus beyond the obvious is the real game and I was somehow learning how to play.

How many times in the past had I looked at a problem and found the outcome to be more valuable than what caused it in the first place? A light bulb began to blink above my head. Isn't how I react to disorder ultimately what will free me from it?

The tougher questions lay beneath the surface: if I didn't survive this, would my life have been everything I'd wanted it to be? Would there be apologies left unsaid? Forgiveness denied? Had I done everything I could to leave the world a little better than it was before I got here?

On the flipside—and perhaps most important—if I survived this, would I make a daily commitment to those same principles?

They removed the cancer early enough and even saved my

kidney. That's the good news. The bad news—if you want to call it that—is that it may return. There are two spots on my other kidney. They, too, might be malignant. That my cancer is a rare, hereditary form increases the likelihood. The doctor says all we can do is watch and wait.

CT scans will likely become a way of life for me, something I'll have to live with for a long time, but I refuse to see them as constant reminders of the deadly intruder lurking within my cell structure. For me, they are reminders of something else, something much more important. They remind me of time, my most priceless commodity. It's not about how much of it I have. It's about how much I do with it.

Living each day like it's your last is like climbing the tallest mountain in the world. It doesn't matter how long you get to look down. Just being able to see it makes every second priceless and every step well worth the trip.

I didn't really know that before. The disease has changed that.

The way I to respond to cancer will reveal its true meaning for me. I have moved past my tragedy and found its significance. The further I have gone, the clearer it has actually become.

Each day is a one-time offer.

~Andrew E. Kaufman

Becoming a Patient

I was first diagnosed with breast cancer fifteen years ago. I was a single parent with two daughters: one away in college and a twelve-year-old at home. I was also in love with the man who is now my husband.

Having been an oncology social worker for fourteen years, I thought I knew a great deal about living with cancer. I was wrong. The diagnosis literally brought me to my knees.

I decided to be treated at the hospital that had long been my professional home. I wondered whether it was fair to ask my friends to be my caregivers. With their words: "I can't stand taking care of you, but I would hate it more if anyone else were," and "If we can't take care of each other, what good are we in this world?" I knew that it was the right decision.

Those of us who work in oncology make a pact with the gods. If we devote our lives to taking care of others, our own lives, and those of people whom we love, will be protected. Intellectually, we know that it's not so, but in our hearts, the contract is sealed.

My diagnosis shattered any magical thinking that lingered. In spite of my relative youth, forty-four, and excellent health, something really bad had happened. For several weeks, I said nothing to my patients, rationalizing that they would be upset by the news. The truth was, I couldn't bear to say it out loud.

Eventually, I had to share the news. With almost no exceptions, everyone reacted with genuine affection and empathy. The months that followed transformed my life's work to my own.

Since my diagnosis, I have had great credibility. I have often wondered why anyone previously believed a single word that I uttered. What blind faith my patients once placed in me.

As the years passed, I worried less about a recurrence. I never felt completely safe, but I stopped being constantly afraid. It never occurred to me to worry that I might develop a second primary breast cancer and yet that's what happened in 2005.

There is no literature about how to manage cancer a second time while continuing to work as an oncology social worker, being married to an oncologist in the same practice, and dealing with collegial and patient relationships that become traumatized.

Unlike the first time, the diagnosis exploded. My yearly mammogram revealed an area of concern that would require a core biopsy.

My situation complicated matters with my patients. For better or for worse, I knew that I had become a role model of how to live with cancer. Watching me, healthy and strong and happy, had given hope to many women newly diagnosed. Unlike 1993, when I wondered if I would ever stop crying, this second time, I was dry-eyed. There was work to be done.

At the same time, I felt very vulnerable, aware of my mortal fragility, and mourned even the small possibility of ever living in blissful denial. I was achingly aware of the wonder, richness, and love of my life, and the possibility that cancer could steal it from me too soon. I was overwhelmed with sorrow and regret for what it could do to my husband, my daughters, my family, my friends, and my colleagues.

My husband, Chief of Oncology at our hospital, was put in a more public and vulnerable position than he would have ever chosen. When patients asked him, "If I were your wife, what would you tell me to do?" the question took on an entirely different meaning. As my diagnosis was revealed, many wondered, "If they could not even protect Hester, what will happen to me?"

Surgery was scheduled for the following week. Most of my

patients were wonderful. Unfortunately, a few were not. One woman, in the midst of a medical crisis herself, literally jumped from her chair to shake her fist at me: "How dare you leave me now? How dare you have cancer again?"

The primary physical aftermath of this surgery is fatigue not pain, so, when I was awake, I generally felt pretty well. My younger daughter stayed a week, and was then relieved by her older sister who stayed the second. We had not had that kind of time together for years, and it was wonderful.

The most difficult clinical interactions were around privacy and my insistence that I not be metaphorically swallowed up by my patients. I had been living "cancer on a pedestal" and "cancer in a fishbowl." There was tremendous pressure, mostly self-imposed, to look as well as possible every day. Buying a good wig helped; having a consult with the make-up maven helped more.

I was surprised by how much I hated being bald; I felt ugly, vulnerable, and very public. A few days after shaving my head in anticipation of the hair loss, I went with my family to a local ice cream stand. I was wearing a hat, feeling terribly self-conscious, when I overheard someone nearby say, "Oh, look; she must have cancer." I fled to the car. I felt humiliated and shamed. After all these years of being the cancer professional, I could not bear being the public patient. And yet I had to be.

Getting dressed became a clinical decision. I had to consider the day's appointments to figure out what I could wear on my head. I could not imagine walking into our waiting room, introducing myself to a newly diagnosed breast cancer patient and having her see, in one horrified instant that I, too, was on chemotherapy. Once my eyebrows and eyelashes were gone, it was even worse. Surprisingly, given the hype about the improvement around symptom control during chemotherapy, this course was much more difficult than the one I endured in 1993.

I took a few days off during the course of chemotherapy, but was almost always at work, even though I felt constantly nauseated. Each morning began with my husband's bedside delivery of tea and saltines. Many days, I forced myself to get to the gym, per my usual routine, and found that the workout and the camaraderie improved my psychological, if not my physical, outlook. I survived at work on warm ginger ale, a holdover from childhood.

Finally, with two weekly treatments to go, I accompanied my husband on a trip to Switzerland where he was giving a talk. He, my doctor, and my nurse practically pushed me onto that airplane; I was too exhausted to imagine such an undertaking.

"You can sleep just as well in Geneva," they told me, and they were right. Those few days were the beginning of my recovery. Sitting by the lake, looking at the Alps, I remembered the beauties and the possibilities of the world. I even began to believe that I could rejoin it.

And now, three years later, I feel strong again, healthy, and happy. Again, I am slipping into less fear and more trust with my health, in spite of the daily reminders that it could always happen again.

~Hester Hill Schnipper, LICSW, BCD, OSW-C

Numb

It was just another day in middle school—joking around, making fun of kids, and disrupting classes. Math was the last one of the day and most kids found it to be a joke because the teacher had no control over our behavior and we exploited that.

In the middle of class, my friend Sam handed me a letter with my name on it. I was certain I was in trouble—again. That was my daily routine: getting a letter from one of my teachers, being sent to the office, getting detention or even suspended.

The letter was written by my mother, informing the teacher that my father had cancer and to please be more lenient with me in class. I raced out of the classroom, crying. All of the kids thought I was trying to disrupt things, as usual, and my teacher came running after me, yelling for me to come back.

He caught me in the hallway and told me to calm down. I told him what the letter said and I asked him if he had read it too. He reluctantly said yes and kindly offered to take me to the office, where my mother was waiting to pick me up.

I was anxious the rest of the day as I waited for my father to show up. Finally, in the evening, he arrived in his black Volkswagen Beetle, surprised to find me waiting for him in front of my mom's apartment building.

For the next hour, we discussed how to go about things, but I didn't feel like much of a participant. The conversation was more at me than with me. My parents were doing their best to relieve my stress, but every word they spoke corresponded with cancer. They asked me if I had any questions but I was too numb to say a word. That single hour was the most serious, real moment I had ever spent in my thirteen-year-old life.

After that, everything changed.

As my father's sickness became a lifestyle, it affected my average day. I would leave school but not find him there to pick me up. I would call to play catch or go for a drive, but he would be too tired. I would go days without seeing him. If I brought up cancer, he would shut down, and if I brought up an interesting topic, he would loosely listen. Our bonding time turned into questions about his possible death, which irritated and scared him. So, we did mindless activities, like watching TV.

One night, at my mom's house, I found out that his cancer had spread to the brain. I immediately ran outside in my shorts even though it was snowy. I had to find my dad and hold him. I ran to his apartment and he was surprised to see me. He acted as if nothing was wrong, and I asked him if the illness had really gotten worse. He told me he was feeling fine, but I knew how sick he was. Days later, his illness became more obvious as he began slurring his words. He had headaches and he was irritable all the time.

Every night before I got in bed I would ask my mom if my dad's condition was "in the status quo." One night, she told me the cancer had spread to his liver. I just cried all night.

Focusing was pretty tough during school. I left class frequently just to think. While my dad was dying, everything I did seemed like it might not last. My father's health seemed short term and my relationship with him was too.

On the day my dad died, my mom came to school and told me it was time. I went to his apartment and watched a man in a bed waiting to die, a man named George who seemed like someone I'd never met before. No one knows if he accepted his death, but my eyes saw a man who was ready.

When it was finally over, I didn't really know how to feel. I was in a state of shock, but mostly I was ready for a new beginning. I was sad, but I was also happy. I was glad my father was out of pain.

I didn't have to deal with the stress of him dying anymore. But, unfortunately, when every single person shared their condolences all it did was make me think about him.

Looking back, I think one of the most depressing days was when we saw our last movie together. I woke up that day knowing it would be the last one. He was getting too skinny and too tired, and he was ready to die. That morning, my mother and I dragged him out of his apartment and took a taxi to the theater.

Constantine was about the devil and death, and made sharing the last movie with my dad very awkward. Most of all, it was sad. Imagine having to say goodbye to your dad for like, forever. The whole time I was just trying to make conversation to get my mind off him dying. But he didn't feel like talking. He was just dying.

The way I am now is confusing. There are some things that I can't think about or I will cry. Thinking about the year that he had cancer mostly does it for me. Sometimes, I see father-son relationships on TV or in the movies and I get pretty sad. However, on a typical day I barely think about him. I do have fears that other loved ones will become ill and I will have to deal with the same process all over again. I also fear that my mother will die and I will have no parents.

Sometimes, I blame things in my life on my dad's passing from cancer. But right now, that whole thing was a brief period in my life that I never want to think about.

~Joseph O'Rourke, age 17

Chicken Soup
of the Soul

Tough

"That's an impressive tumor," my doctor said, showing me the X-ray.

I had hoped the appointment would be quick because even though I coughed all the way through the exam I couldn't really afford the break from work.

He was busy and a little exasperated with me. But my doctor is maddeningly thorough. He checked my lungs, my sinuses, my breath output—all with no conclusion. He mumbled something about ruling out pneumonia but I think he really sent me down for a chest X-ray just to buy some time before he prescribed a tranquilizer and therapy.

After the X-ray, I was left alone in an unused exam room for what seemed like forever. It was dark and eerily quiet outside. I was sure I'd been forgotten. I had mountains of work waiting for me and my frustration grew. I thought about walking out and calling later, but I was so tired and resting in that lonely room wasn't that bad.

The doctor finally came and showed me the X-ray. I couldn't comprehend what I was seeing or what he was saying. He's normally business-like, a little brusque, and sometimes sarcastic, but he was clearly shaken as he pointed to that sponge-like, white mass between my lungs and tried to explain what I was seeing.

That was the first time I heard the phrase, "impressive tumor." Now, I hear it from every doctor when they see the scans, as they introduce themselves and shake my hand. It's like I'm being congratulated for giving a great speech or breaking an Olympic record, while all I've done is accidentally grow a giant, malignant mass around my windpipe.

The other thing I hear repeatedly is that I'm tough.

Even people I barely know say, "You're tough. You'll be fine."

What does that mean? What if I'm not tough? How does anyone know I'm tough enough to survive this? I've decided it's a standard phrase people like to use, like a coach encouraging his star kicker before he goes onto the field. Like if people say it enough, I'll start to believe it and make it come true. My husband, Dave, says they're not kidding.

"Everyone can see how tough you are."

I always thought it would be cool to be tough. I wanted to be that bad girl: rail thin, wearing a black leather jacket and smoking a cigarette outside some punk rock bar. I don't think that's what people mean when they call me tough. Am I tough like stringy beef? Like a gang member from *West Side Story*? Maybe I'm tough like the suitcase the gorilla stomps on in the old commercial.

How does any of that help me survive cancer?

I keep showing up for chemotherapy and do my best to hang on during the three ghastly days after each session. When I'm not sick, I meditate, exercise, and call my friends and family for support. I sleep a lot. I journal. I cry. I don't feel tough.

My beautiful hair began coming out in handfuls. I left embarrassing trails of hair in people's cars and on chair backs. My normal hair bands wouldn't stay put.

I mourned. I fretted. I have always been vain about my hair. After the second treatment, my normally thick hair started looking stringy and greasy. Lots of gray started coming through, but coloring it was out of the question.

So I did it. I took it all off. I shaved my head. It was easier and harder than I thought. I have read over and over that shaving your head is one way to take charge of the treatment process when so much is out of your control. Great advice, but there is not one word written on how physically difficult it is to shave a full head of hair. I have new respect for Army barbers.

I stood in front of the mirror in my pajamas, contemplating how to start. I cut as much as I could reach. I cried as I watched my expensive highlights pile up in the garbage. I took Dave's electric razor and whoosh! Back to front, front to back. I looked like a warrior from *Braveheart*, with strange tufts and bare patches all over my head.

My seventeen-year-old daughter, Jessica, heard the razor and came to see what was happening. I handed it to her and said, "Do the back." Bless her. She did a great job finishing what I had missed.

When she was done, I was bald. I didn't see a freak or a crazy person. I saw me.

I looked tough.

~Liz Elliott

Cancer
Cannot Cripple Love

I was eleven years old when my world came crashing down. It started when my brother tumbled down the stairs, hurting his ankle. We thought he had a sprain, but the tests showed nothing at all. My mom ordered more tests but nobody was worried, especially me. I was more focused on getting ready for my first year of middle school. Surely nothing horrible was happening to my older brother, the one person who has been there for me, as my rock and my friend, from the minute I was born.

I was wrong.

My dad came home from the hospital, sat me down on my bed, and looked me straight in the eye. I bounced up and down on the mattress, waiting for him to say Matthew had a sprained ankle. But those weren't the words I heard.

"Emily, Matthew has cancer. Things are going to be different from now on."

My innocent smile faded because I knew what cancer was. My grandma had it but she survived. I remembered the pictures of her sick, with no hair. I couldn't imagine my brother losing his hair. I loved his hair, along with most of the girls in his grade. As I sat on my bed, a million things flashed through my head. When I pictured Matthew, my hero, in pain, I started to cry.

From that day on, things were never the same.

Chemotherapy was difficult. Matthew was tired and always throwing up. Cancer made Matthew a completely different person. But he stayed strong. He stayed alive. He saw his cancer as nothing more than a really bad cold, so I did, too. It would go away, never to return, and we could go back to our normal lives.

But not so fast. Cancer likes to leave a mark on everyone connected to it.

I came home from school one day, and what a terrible day it had been. My best friend and I had a falling out and she had punched me very hard on the shoulder. Our friendship was over and I knew it. I thought that things could not get worse, but cancer had other things in store.

My mom drove me home and said Matthew had some news for me. I immediately thought he would have to be shipped off to some hospital far, far away and I wouldn't see him for months. But when I saw the look on Matthew's face, it was obvious. I knew it all along. I sat down and just blurted it out.

"They're going to take your leg, aren't they?" My brother looked down and nodded. It was the worst day of my life.

After the amputation, things got rough. The pain was excruciating for Matthew, and it was hard for him to handle. I would wake up to him screaming every night, and I lost a lot of sleep. My friends could not begin to understand what I was going through and I had no desire to talk to kids in the same situation; it would only depress me even more. So I decided not to deal with it. Instead, I would focus on silly school dramas, just like every preteen should.

Finally, after many sidetracks (including him breaking the top of his amputated leg), Matthew headed into remission. I wish I could say I was ecstatic, thrilled, and excited. But I was numb. It was the first good news in a long time. The only thing I did absorb was that I had my brother back.

Things slowly returned to normal. Matthew was once again complaining about school, people stopped spreading rumors that he was going to die, and I was able to wave away the school dramas that had occupied too much of my energy.

Instead, I looked forward to my cruise to Mexico with my grandparents and my best friend, Pilar, who was like my sister. The cruise started out great, and we were having a very memorable time together. The day after we left was the day Matthew had to get his scans to see if the cancer had returned.

It was December 22nd, 2006.

The second I saw the look in my grandpa's eyes, I knew it was back. Pilar and I spent the whole day crying and holding each other.

I was more ready for it the second time. Matthew and Dad were home even less than before so I turned my attention to my best guy friend to ease the pain I felt in their absence. I also tried to visit as much as possible, but getting to know everyone in the hospital depressed me. I never felt good being a regular.

My mom and dad were eventually faced with a tough decision. A stem cell transplant could save my brother's life, but it could also end it. A bone marrow transplant was another option (and I was to be the donor), but his chances of relapsing were greater.

One day it was to be the bone marrow, the next the stem cell, the next neither, and so on. By the time I was in eighth grade, and hating it, they had settled on the stem cell transplant, which would mean around a month in the hospital for Matthew, receiving stem cells into his bloodstream. I was incredibly nervous, especially when my mom told me about the chances of survival.

All the hugs of support from kids in my grade could not help how scared I was. Throughout the school trip I was stuck on, I was miserable and my friends drew away from me. I kept thinking about my brother, stuck in the hospital.

A few days after Thanksgiving, Matthew was released from the hospital, in full remission. After missing his freshman and sophomore year and half his junior year, he returned to school to complete everything all at once. It was great to have him back, even if I still had to see him in a wheelchair. It just felt right. I could finally leave my numb and cold stage behind and become a typical teenage girl.

When I look back, I remember the emotional sidetracks. Nobody ever asked me how I was doing. It was always how Matthew was, or my mom or dad. But never me.

I was the messenger. But sometimes, someone would get the message. After Matthew was officially in remission, my best guy friend came up to me, put his hand on my shoulder, and told me that he was glad I was okay.

And it was true. I was okay. I am okay. I have overcome being neglected.

I am finally ready for high school.

~Emily Beaver, age 14

How Do I Say This?

D ear Parents of Incoming Fourth Graders,

I hope that summer's end finds you well rested and excited to begin a new school year.

Well rested? Who am I kidding? I haven't slept in a week.

I'm really looking forward to getting off to a good start with your kids and I'm very excited to meet with you and your child. But first, I would like to update you on some of the events that have recently transpired in my life and describe how they may affect the experiences of your children at school this year.

What a mouthful. Enough pleasantries, better just say it. IT? Can I say IT without them calling school to withdraw their kids?
You're not a serial killer. You're a teacher, and a darn good one, so teach.

I have recently been diagnosed with Stage IV Hodgkin's Lymphoma, a relatively rare cancer of the lymphatic system, discovered after a routine physical this summer. In the coming months, I will be undergoing twelve cycles of ABVD chemotherapy with the possibility of radiation treatment to follow.

Boy, I'd hate to be a parent receiving this letter. Just what a new school year needs—more stress. And what about the kids? I'm sure this isn't how they've pictured their return to the classroom. I can hear it already:

"Watch out! Here he comes! He looks weird! Don't let him touch you!"

And, worst of all, "My grandpa died of cancer. Is my teacher gonna die?"

I want to assure all of you that I have surrounded myself with the very best team of Lymphoma specialists and they assure me that my prognosis looks very good.

Yeah, and do I have that in writing anywhere?

Our school administration has been very receptive to my new situation and has very kindly offered to support me in any way I need.

That's good because two months after getting married would be a heck of a time to lose my job. I hope they're serious about supporting me in any way I need.

To that end, they will be hiring an assistant to help me in the classroom on days when I'm not feeling well enough to come to school.

Hopefully, there won't be too many days like that. Oh my god, I could miss weeks at a time. I hope they'll get someone good.

Those of you whose children I've taught in the past will probably guess that I will be completely open with the students in sharing my experience.

To a point. They don't need to know the really bad stuff. Is there going to be really bad stuff? How do I share that without sharing too much?

(Of course, I will do this in an age-appropriate manner.)

I see this as one of life's great "teachable moments" and I don't intend to squander it.

What if these parents don't buy it? Like, who needs a sick teacher hanging out with my kid every day? What if there's an uproar and it spreads?

I need to tread carefully. Perhaps I should be less cavalier about it.

I cannot imagine a better place to be during the months ahead. The doctors assure me that Hodgkin's Disease has a very high survival rate, and I am confident that the numbers are on my side. I have every intention of setting a good example for your kids. So, what I may lack in fortune, I'll make up for in fight.

I wonder if my hair will fall out. I wonder how fast.

"Hey, watch it, will ya? You're getting hair all over my homework!"

At least my wife can't stop me from shaving my head! This is my chance to look like a professional soccer player! A skinny, nauseous, soccer player, but anyway, I've always wanted to have something in common with Lance.

I count myself lucky to teach at a school with such a close-knit, supportive community of teachers, students, and parents.

How am I going to make it through this entire year?

How long can I keep a brave face on?

If I can't hack it, what will that mean for all of us?

I know that different families may handle news like this differently. I invite you all to initiate dialogues with your children so that they will have some prior knowledge of cancer when I explain it to them at school. If you have any questions about methods or details, please feel free to call me at home.

Which kids do I have this year? I'll have to check the list. Certain kids might not be able to deal with their teacher going through this. Changes might need to be made.

I want to thank all of you in advance for your patience and understanding.

I look forward to seeing you in school.

I look forward to writing you my next letter, announcing I am cancer-free.

Fondly,

And terrified,

~Benjamin Schwartz

Cancer Sucks

'm your average teenage girl. I like to shop, hang out with friends, play sports, fight with my parents, and check out boys—all that good teenage stuff.

Besides that, I'm not average, and hope to never be. Last year, I was diagnosed with a cancerous brain tumor. And since then, my life has changed and never will be the same.

Saturday, January 12th.

I felt like I was going to throw up, but I couldn't get out of bed. Finally, I made it to the bathroom. My parents took me to the clinic. I was given a shot and sent home.

Sunday, I went to church and did my homework.

Monday, I felt sick again so I didn't eat breakfast. But I'm serious about school, and my exams were coming up so I wasn't going to let a headache and a bad stomach stop me.

While walking home with my boyfriend, I felt extremely dizzy. I fell into a puddle. I couldn't walk without help so Peter let me place my head on his chest as he walked backwards all the way home, which was actually quite a feat.

My mother took me immediately to our family doctor. When I stepped off the examining table, I had to feel around for the ground with my foot before I could step down and even then I felt terribly off balance.

At the hospital, I was placed inside an MRI machine that made the loudest, most awful noises I'd ever heard. I wasn't allowed to move at all.

Hours later, my doctor arrived and asked to see my parents out in the hallway. This may work with younger children, but I was fifteen years old and I knew it could only be bad news, even though I never thought it was going to be anything too terrible.

My parents said I had a brain tumor. I wasn't scared or worried and I wanted them to know that right away so I just chuckled and smiled and said okay.

Six days later, I had my operation. The last thing I remember was a cold room with a big table.

The next day, after eleven hours of surgery, I couldn't move. I must've been in pretty bad shape, judging by the looks of my family. My entire face was severely swollen from lying on my stomach during surgery and I was in immense pain.

That's when I saw my father cry—my father, who has always been my inspiration, the man I've always looked up to as my rock, who I'd never seen in a weak moment, much less crying. He was pacing as the tears fell from his face and I knew he didn't want me to see him so torn apart. Only at that moment did I cry for the first time.

When I got home a week later, I couldn't move my neck or return to school. I sat at home for weeks, occupying myself with television and trying to move my neck.

I was never alone for long. I had visitors—school friends, coaches, friends of my parents, parents of my friends—it seemed like everyone was sending cards and coming over. I had never known that so many people cared for me. I also received hundreds of cards from people I didn't even know and that amazed me.

Finally, I went back to school and was overwhelmed by the work. But my teachers worked through it with me.

A month later, I started radiation and chemo. I had to lie on my stomach with my head strapped tightly to the table. This was uncomfortable and painful. The radiation didn't hurt, but it smelled.

My dislike for the smell grew so bad that just entering the building could nauseate me.

I also started losing my hair. At first, it fell out in small clumps and I tried with all my might not to think about it. But one night, after growing so tired of it falling out, I started gently pulling. Five minutes later, my entire hairline was pushed back at least four inches.

The next day, more and more fell out. I was so torn up I asked my father to shave my head. I knew he could do it because he's strong-willed and he's been shaving his own head for years. But I couldn't stand the sight of my hair falling to the ground and I asked him to stop. I cried and couldn't breathe. My dad held me and calmed me down. That marked the second time I had cried. Ten minutes later, he finished my head.

I went to school the next day, wearing a hat. I didn't let anyone see my "new look" unless it was a close friend or the occasional person who asked. I'm far from being shy. I'm loud, opinionated, and I like to think I'm fun. But losing something that's such a part of me, like my hair, made me much less confident.

I gradually got used to my new head but hated the way it looked without being tan. Since our family was about to go on our annual vacation to Florida I would have a chance to tan my new, hairless head.

At first, I was self-conscious because of the large scar on the back of my head. But gradually, I convinced myself that I was going to be me no matter what I looked like.

Then, someone on the beach told me I was beautiful. Not because of my looks but because of how I never seemed to care about any kind of troubles and just lived my life. That week, I began to get my confidence back. I realized that my self-assuredness should never come from how I look, but from how I feel inside, from knowing who I am and loving myself. I returned to school and never wore a hat again.

I didn't want to be treated like a cancer patient anymore. I went out for the softball team and made varsity. Softball is a huge part of my life. I've played since I was in second grade. It's one of the things I love most.

I was part of a team and I wasn't treated specially because I had cancer. I had to miss some practices and a game or two because of treatments but it was all worth it. I was on the front page of our newspaper and even in *Sports Illustrated*. People thought I was doing something brave or special, but to me it just felt normal.

I didn't understand why I was getting so much publicity for just being me and doing what I do all the time. So, my parents explained inspiration to me.

One time in the radiation room, I was given a button that read "Cancer Sucks."

Personally, I think that's the best way to look at it. Cancer does suck, and the sooner you accept that, the sooner you can realize that no matter how much it sucks you have to deal with it, and that you might as well deal with it with a smile.

~Emmarie Truman, age 16

From Tiara to Tumor to Team

Three months after being crowned Homecoming Princess in her sophomore year of high school, our fifteen-year-old daughter, Emmarie, was diagnosed with brain cancer.

Our family had always been blessed with extremely good health and all three of our girls were athletes, so hearing the words "brain tumor" seemed too surreal to believe. I felt like I was underwater and I was watching the scene unfold around me in slow motion. The doctor had tears in her eyes. I remember my husband Allen saying, "Well, we've just got to turn it over to the Lord now." We all held hands and prayed for courage before telling Emmarie the news.

They called it a medulloblastoma tumor and although we had hoped to hear the beautiful B word—benign—the tumor turned out to be much more vascular, aggressive, and fast-growing than the neurosurgeons had originally thought.

When they said it was the size of a small lemon, I thought of that old line, "When life gives you a lemon, make lemonade." But at that moment, I couldn't imagine how anything good could possibly come from this situation. My dad had given me a stone carving for my last birthday with the inscription, "And we know that in all things God works for the good of those that love Him"(Romans 8:28). We had to move forward in blind faith that this lemon was in God's hands, and that if any lemonade was to be made from this, then God was in charge of making it!

In order to kill off any renegade cancer cells that might have still been lurking anywhere in Emmarie's brain, spine, or central nervous system after the surgery she required fourteen months of radiation and chemotherapy, continuing deep into her junior year of high school. We wondered how she would cope. Being fifteen is tough enough, in the best of circumstances, without throwing cancer into the mix.

Emmarie, like the rest of us, learned that life isn't predictable. It takes strange twists and turns. One minute you're on top of the world, a star, wearing a sparkling tiara on a head full of hair. The next you're trading in your star for a scar with a single strand of hair left to cover it.

Emme decided not to focus on the scar or the cancer, for that matter. She began to tell people "I used to have cancer, but I beat it." I marveled at that.

She decided to make the most of her new look, quit wearing hats, and went to school bald. She hated the stares from people but she decided to make it work in her favor. She thought, "If I can be myself, without hair, then I'll definitely be stronger and able to tackle anything when this is over." She decided to focus outward instead of inward. I marveled at that, too.

Only two months after discovering her brain tumor, Emme tried out for the varsity softball team and made it! Her coach was impressed with her persistence and winning spirit.

We focused on our many blessings. We live in an era when so much good cancer research is happening. Forty years ago, Emme would have had only a ten percent survival rate. Now, she has an eighty-five percent chance.

Most of all, we focused on our faith, family, and friends. Relatives and neighbors popped in with food, cards, and beautiful words of hope. Emmarie's friends made posters and brought her funny wigs and gag gifts. We were especially blessed to have so many people praying for Emme, from all over this country and other parts of the world.

Oh don't get me wrong. There are hard days, times when spirits droop, attitudes suffer and she gets "sick of being sick." But overall, Emmarie is fighting a good fight and learning to take life one step at a time. I was proud of her that night last fall when she walked out on that football field, crowned Homecoming Princess, but that was nothing compared to how proud I am now to be Emmarie's mom. Sometimes it takes a scar or two to make a "star" truly shine.

~Elaine Truman

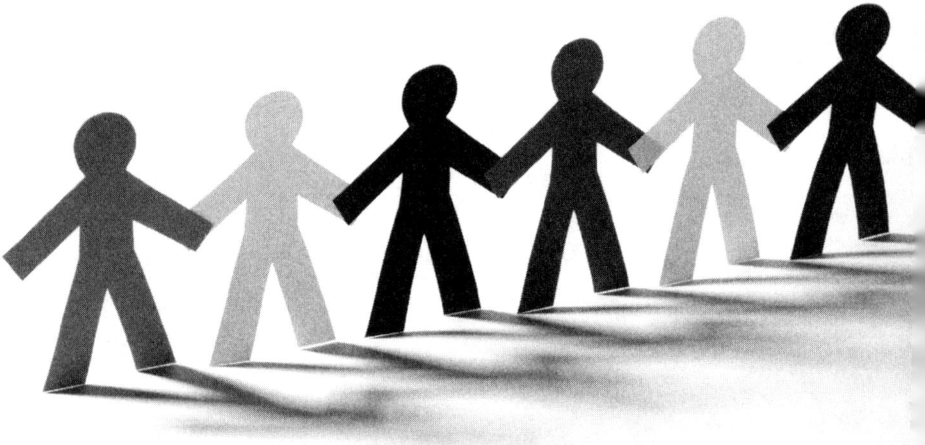

The Cancer Book

Not So Soon

I know God will not give me anything I can't handle.
I just wish that He didn't trust me so much.

~Mother Teresa

Changing the World

"Am I gonna die while I'm still a kid?"

The air was sucked out of my lungs by that unexpected and heartbreaking question from our six-year-old daughter, Sarah. I had no idea what had been going through her sweet, bald head as she serenely spooned Cheerios into her mouth, blissfully unaware of the small drop of milk festooning her chin.

Trying to keep my composure, I replied, "How do you feel about that, Sarah?"

She said softly, "I'd prefer to live."

I couldn't help think of an e-mail I'd received from a woman who also has a daughter with Stage IV neuroblastoma which said, "I catch myself grieving for her while she's still here."

Sarah interrupted my thoughts.

"Mom, when I die will you please put my blankey in the grave with me?"

I froze for a second and did my best to calm my voice before asking, "Is that what you want, Sarah?"

"Yup," she replied.

Sarah's face was pale and peeling from the treatment but her eyes were bright and merry as she crawled onto my lap for our traditional post-breakfast snuggle. Once I'd wrapped her blankey around her, we sat quietly in our mother/daughter cocoon, the tears running down my face as I thought how desperately I would miss those moments if the day came when cancer stole her away.

I couldn't help but wonder. Is this some kind of extended goodbye? If Sarah lives a long life, I will be so grateful. But if she dies so young, while she can still fit into my lap, I will still be thankful for the short time we've had.

I wonder if the symptoms she's been experiencing lately are the beginning of the end or nothing at all. It's the endless uncertainty that's so difficult—waiting for the phone to ring and a doctor's words to shatter our world, receiving e-mails from other parents who are hurting, reading books about cancer and stories on websites of other children who have died from neuroblastoma—and not knowing how long our goodbye might be.

All I want is for Sarah to live long enough to truly taste life, to grow tall and have hair long enough to put into pigtails, to date, to learn the art of teenage eye-rolling and to go to college. All I want is for my daughter to live. And yet, I am so afraid that the morning will come when she won't be here and that so many clouds will cover my heart that I will never again see the sun. But I also know that she could survive for many years. It's a strange place to be, dreading the fear and pain of the future while embracing the hope and joy of each memory we make.

We experienced one of those moments when Sarah was in the hospital on Halloween, receiving chemo, and the staff organized trick-or-treating for the few kids well enough to participate. Sarah donned a SpongeBob outfit and cheerily took off down the hall, swinging her orange bucket with great enthusiasm. She was a contented compatriot in a hall full of heroes—brave, battle-worn children accompanied by compassionate nurses, willing to risk having their hearts broken every time they came to work.

As I watched my small, bald SpongeBob, I was thankful for the privilege of being with my daughter for such a special but ordinary moment.

After the trick-or-treaters collected their candy, Sarah suddenly announced wearily from behind her mask, "Mommy, my steam just ran out!"

I said, "That's okay, honey. I'll just pick you up and carry you."

As I helped Sarah back into her hospital bed, I couldn't help but question if a time might come when she would leave that hospital room and go away to a place where there is no cancer, no bald children and no sound of small hearts breaking. I thought about a day when Sarah "SpongeBob" Smith might say, "My steam ran out," and God would respond, "That's okay, Sarah. I'll just pick you up and carry you."

I'd rather Sarah not fly to that place anytime soon, but I'm so glad that whenever her time comes, she'll be ready. The truth is, during her cancer treatment, our roles have been reversed. She's become the teacher and I have become the student. I've seen her go through chemo, surgeries, a bone marrow transplant, and radiation, and more pain, tears, and sadness than any mother's heart can bear. And yet I've seen her get up in the morning, fuss over her little animals, smile at me, snuggle in my lap, and exhibit incredible strength and joy as she unflinchingly faces each scary moment.

• • •

And now, six years later, at the age of thirteen, Sarah is well.

When she was diagnosed, her chances of surviving five years were twenty percent. But I guess she didn't get the memo. Sarah lives life large, with the kind of zest and appreciation for each day that only someone who has come so close to death can truly understand. Her wonderful health is due to prayer, great doctors, and the modern miracle of blood transfusions.

When chemo turned her into a pale and listless shadow of herself, it took only one transfusion for Sarah's cheeks to blossom and for her to jump off her bed and back into life. In the weeks after her immune system had been completely wiped out by intensive chemo in preparation for her bone marrow transplant, she would have died many times over without the numerous transfusions of platelets and red blood cells she received.

Without those transfusions, my daughter would be dead. Without them, the answer to "Am I going to die when I'm a kid?" would have been "Yes."

•••

Years ago, while sitting in the nuclear medicine waiting room as Sarah changed into a gown, I described to a woman dealing with her own cancer what my daughter was going through. As I mentioned each thing on the list, I could see her sadness grow at the thought of a small child having to endure so much.

Suddenly, we heard the unmistakable sound of Sarah's sweet, small voice. The lady was incredulous as she whispered, "I just can't believe your daughter is singing!"

The chairs around us were filled with people of all ages, their heads bent low, each of them disheartened by somber thoughts and anxious realities. One by one, I saw their heads rise as they heard Sarah singing. The fear on their faces was temporarily replaced with involuntary smiles. It was as if a tidal wave of sunshine had swept the room.

Sarah gave them a little infusion of courage and joy as they submitted their bodies to the machines that would spell out life or death. She gave them a reason to smile.

Sarah has often told me, "Mommy, I was born to make people smile."

Living with cancer has allowed Sarah to fulfill her mission in a greater way than she could have ever imagined. And she's changing the world for me every day that she lives.

My teacher is my child. My child is my life. May our goodbye never come.

~Becky Campbell Smith

12

The Wrong Answer

As the kids in my fifth-grade class worked on their math journals, the telephone rang. I needed to dismiss them in a few minutes. My wife, Rhonda, was on the phone and she said something neither of us had expected.

"The biopsy report came back as cancerous."

I heard the word cancer and stared at my students, huddled over their books, seeking the answers to multiplication problems. Little did they know that on the other end of the phone was someone who just realized she was about to face the battle of her life—in fact, the battle for life itself—and she was telling their teacher that his family's life was about to change forever.

The students' answers were either right or wrong. Cancer seemed, in my mind, in that moment, to be the wrong answer to a question I hadn't even dared ask.

Did the doctors really have this right? Rhonda's family had no known history of breast cancer. How could this diagnosis be true?

The ten- and eleven-year-old children sitting at their desks, who knew nothing of what raced through my mind, glanced anxiously at the clock as time for music class came closer. I pulled the phone away from my head and dismissed them. They left the way kids often do—the way I wish I could relearn—leaving their problems behind and moving on.

Once my class was gone, I felt free to ask specifics. As Rhonda began describing what little she knew from her phone conversation with the surgeon, I jotted down quick notes.

I said "I love you," and hung up the phone.

For a few moments, I sat, stunned, then methodically typed some search terms into my computer and found that what Rhonda mentioned indicated a cancer that had been caught early and was very treatable, an indication we later found out was totally incorrect.

Many thoughts crowded my mind. How does one respond to a spouse who has breast cancer? My own mom had battled breast cancer twice and was doing well. I had every reason to believe the same would be true for Rhonda. But, what exactly should I do? When? And, how?

I knew I would be unable to finish the day at school, so I made arrangements to have my class covered for the remainder of the day.

The drive home was long. My mind jumped from one confusing thought to another. When I entered our home, Rhonda and I hugged each other and got caught up on who had been contacted thus far about the diagnosis.

Our middle son, Michael, then fourteen and home-schooled, wondered why I was home early. I listened as Rhonda told him she had been diagnosed with breast cancer. He gave no verbal hints about what he thought. I wonder exactly what goes through a teenage boy's mind when he hears this kind of thing from his own mother.

Jonathon, then sixteen and a junior in high school, came home from school a bit later, and I told him the news, offering as Rhonda had with Michael the assurance that the cancer had been caught early and was therefore very treatable.

That night, Rhonda called Bethany, our ten-year-old daughter, over to the couch, and as Bethany sat on her lap Rhonda told her she had been diagnosed with cancer. I had expected Bethany's reaction to be one of confusion, uncertainty as to what cancer even was. Instead, she hugged her mom tightly and burst into tears. "What if you die?" she said between sobs.

It wasn't easy to watch such a young child grapple with the idea of losing one of her parents. With what turned out to be false hope, Rhonda reassured her that the cancer had been caught early and would be easily treated.

The following day at school, I stood before one of my classes and wondered what I could really say to a room full of fifth-graders. The day before, I had simply said my wife was not feeling well and I needed to go home—more than an understatement, I guess. What could they really understand about what was happening?

From the tone of my voice and the look on my face it was obvious to them that something was going on. Everything about me probably screamed, "Something is going on!"

And, so I began. I told them my wife had breast cancer and that I would probably be missing a lot of school. They were quiet. Very quiet. Like my own daughter, they knew all too well what the prospect of cancer meant.

Suddenly, my "other children" had joined my changing world. They had become part of this journey called cancer. It stayed quiet until one boy's hand went up.

"My grandpa had cancer," he declared.

"My uncle had cancer," another said.

Some of their stories were of family members who had survived cancer, while some mentioned those who had not. None of the kids seemed to have any desire to elicit fear or morbidity. Instead, their stories were an attempt to make a connection, to bring meaning in the only way they knew how, by relating what they knew of cancer, themselves. It was their way of saying they might not understand everything, but they empathized with my family and me.

One boy's statement as he left for the day still rings in my ear. With his backpack slung over his shoulder, he turned back to me as he neared the exit door.

"I'm sorry about what happened."

His tone of voice was pure and said that he was truly sorry, that he shared this deep hurt in his own heart. This was probably one of the purest forms of compassion I've ever heard, and it came not from another adult or a doctor or nurse, but from a child—a child who sensed my pain and with a few words showed how much he cared.

~Daniel Burns

13

What Makes You Smile?

"Who wants to share what they wished for?" Lam asks.

Every arm in the roomful of children flies up. Support Director Gary Lam points to Andrew, a cherubic six-year-old boy with curly brown hair.

"Swimming with the dolphins!" Andrew calls out, beaming.

Several dozen other campers bounce up and down, eager to share similar experiences.

"Meeting Mickey," cries Jordan.

"I got a shopping spree in a toy store!" says Kendall.

After each wish is revealed, moans of envy echo around the room.

"What other good things have happened because you have cancer?"

An older boy across the circle, about eleven years old, raises his hand.

"Being sick has brought my family closer together. We spend way more time now doing fun stuff."

"If I never went to Children's Hospital," a nine-year-old girl, wearing a pink bandana to cover her bald head, says next, "I never woulda met my best friend!" She squeezes the hand of the pig-tailed girl in a matching bandana, seated next to her.

"I have a new appreciation for life," says Jake, a counselor and former camper, now in his early twenties. "I've crammed more experiences into the last five years than most people have in their lifetime."

Jake is not only the guitar-playing comedian all the campers worship. He's also survived the same battle they are currently fighting.

Lam nods appreciatively. "What would you say is the best thing about cancer?"

Every hand flies up into the air again and Matthew, a mischievous ten-year-old with shaggy blond hair, is chosen. He smirks, and announces proudly, "The best part is getting to look Cancer in the face and say 'Ha Ha. Beat You!'" Everyone laughs.

Seven-year-old Ella, who has been waving her arm frantically for the past few minutes, can't contain herself a moment longer. "The best part about cancer is getting to come to camp!" she squeals, before clamping a hand over her mouth sheepishly.

Ella is referring to Camp Goodtimes—a pediatric oncology camp nestled in the University of British Columbia Research Forest in Maple Ridge, British Columbia. It could easily rival Disneyland for the title of "Happiest Place on Earth."

My first encounter with Camp Goodtimes came four years ago after reading a story in *Chicken Soup for the Volunteer's Soul*, which inspired me to go see the magic for myself. I've been changed ever since.

The feather-light little girl snuggled on my lap shifts her weight slightly and jars my attention back to the room. Dani has been listening intently to the discussion going on around her without actively participating. It's hard to believe this sweet girl is the same sad, sick-looking child who stormed into my cabin on the first day, furious with the world, and anything but a happy camper.

"The sickest kid in camp," a fellow volunteer had warned me. "So let's not let it stop her from having the time of her life." Dani had barely spoken a word the first few days but was silently soaking it all in, and soon began thriving.

Gary Lam circles the room, handing each child a small square of paper and instructing them to write down or draw a picture of something that brings a smile to their face.

Dani furrows her eyebrows and sucks on the end of her marker; then she flops on her tummy and swaps the marker for a pink crayon, and begins printing letters carefully.

"Do you need help thinking of something?" I whisper nervously.

The poor kid has been through so much in the past year, battling treatments and brain surgeries. What could she possibly have to smile about?

She shakes her head at me impatiently, as I'm obviously interrupting her thoughts.

I glance around the circle at Andrew, Ella, Matthew, and all the other new members of my extended camp family. It's going to be heartbreaking to say goodbye in a matter of days. As magical as these precious weeks of summer are, the frustrating part is leaving this enchanted forest behind and returning to reality, where well-meaning friends just don't realize that the cure rate for childhood cancer is actually quite high and that many of the campers will survive and return as counselors.

"You must have had the most depressing time with all those dying kids."

I reflect on the summer's activities. Kayaking through the early morning mist. Baking cookies in our pajamas. Water fights of epic proportions. Breaking into spontaneous song and dance whenever the desire struck.

"Now it's time to share our smiles with the rest of the world," Gary informs the kids. My campers follow me down a gravel path to the lake, holding hands and clutching strings with dozens of balloons dancing in the breeze and bonking our heads with rubbery thuds.

We kneel on the creaky dock and begin the countdown:

"3.....2.....1!"

Dozens of balloons with paper messages attached dancing in the breeze and bonking our heads... we release the balloons—and our optimistic thoughts—up into the sky and out into the universe, watching as they slowly float up, up and away.

"Blow!" Gary yells.

We huff and puff and watch the colorful spheres as they finally disappear from sight. As I survey the young crowd craning their necks for a final glimpse, I marvel at Gary's ability to take a bunch of sick kids and turn a discussion of childhood cancer into such a positive experience. No one was thinking of the hard times. No one was wondering who would be back next summer and who wouldn't.

Dani glances up at me and grins. Just moments earlier, before she had carefully folded her paper in half, sealing her message inside, she'd quickly flashed the paper open to give me a peek.

In bold pink writing, her message simply said: "I Smile Because I'm Alive."

~Cassie Silva

14

Chicken Soup
for the Soul

The Numbers to Live By

100,000,000,000 good cells
10,000 bad ones
Like goblins eating my life away.

7 slender needles puncture me
1 per day
Like a pincushion I am.

1,200 milligrams of deadly yellow liquid
2 big bags full
Like poison in my veins.

100 times a day I'm scared
100 times for what lies ahead
Like a prisoner in my own body.

86 pills swallowed in a week
60 in a single day
Like killers of bad and good.

10,000,000 strands of hair in
1,000,000 strands out
Like a dog, I'm constantly shedding.

10 spinal taps endured
6 more yet to happen
Like a maple tree every three months.

1,100 for a blood count means school for the day
500 means I'm home
Like dictators the numbers rule my life.

100 times a day I ask, "Why me?"
100 times I get no response
Like screams from a roller coaster left unanswered.

130 weeks of pure torture
39 are now history
Like the blink of an eye in slow motion.

100's of people I've met on the way
6 make me better
Like personal guardian angels.

10 sets of numbers to live by,
1 disease called cancer,
Like a pop quiz, it comes out of nowhere.

8 letters in leukemia,
But only 5 in cured.

~Nisha Drummond, age 12

The Catheter

"Have you urinated yet?"

"Nope. I've been trying, but it hasn't happened yet."

"If you don't go by 6 A.M. we're going to have to put a catheter in."

This unpleasant exchange took place shortly after my thyroidectomy, the treatment for my thyroid cancer. I was fifteen, no longer a child but not quite a man either.

After the surgery, my eyelids were still heavy from the anesthesia, feeling like cinder blocks were holding them closed. I could only open my eyes for a split second, enough to take in the surroundings and get a quick snapshot of what was happening as they moved me from post-op to my hospital room.

The Lakers game was on television. The lights were dim. It's always dark when I get out of surgery. The curtain was pulled, separating me from my roommate. My parents were outside in the hallway with Uncle Mike and Aunt Mary.

I was starting to feel nauseous from the anesthesia. I yelled for help, but the tray didn't make it into my hands in time. I didn't vomit much, since I hadn't eaten in sixteen hours, but there was enough to make a mess of my gown and the bed sheets. The nurse was apparently too busy to get me a new gown or new sheets, so I was forced to wallow in the disgusting odor.

My roommate was having his own issues, something to do with his kidneys. He had a different nurse than me. I caught a glimpse of her as she walked past my bed to get to his. She strutted like she was the most important person in the world, or at least in the hospital.

I didn't start paying attention until the tension of the conversation behind the curtain became palpable.

"I'm going to have to put a catheter in."

"NOOOOOOOOOO!"

"I'm going to use lubricant and try to make it hurt as little as possible."

"Please, no. Just give me one more chance."

"I'm sorry."

What followed were guttural grunts and screams coming from both nurse and patient. While I had resigned myself to sleeping in my own vomit, I vowed to do everything in my power to never ever have a catheter.

Hours later, after being moved to a private room, the nursing supervisor made sure I was cleaned up and had received an apology from my nurse. It was an essentially insincere apology, followed by the threat of a catheter. I had about four hours to urinate or else I feared she would follow through with her threat.

My mom spent the night in the room with me. She had heard the exchange in the other room between the kidney patient and the other nurse and had seen how afraid I was, and naturally she wanted to help. Neither one of us slept very much. We had no idea what to really do in order to avoid the dreaded catheter.

My mother bumped into a resident in the cafeteria while she was getting coffee, and he suggested rubbing my abdomen above my bladder to help stimulate the urination process. I was open to any and all suggestions, so I let her do it. It was an odd feeling, being fifteen and having my mother rubbing my lower abdomen while I held the container between my legs, trying to pee. I wanted to be grown-up about the whole situation, but I wasn't exactly in any position to take care of myself.

It didn't work, probably because I was so tense about the catheter.

I finally fell asleep, exhausted from the stress of the whole day. The surgeon came through on rounds at about 6:30 A.M. (the mean nurse was late, apparently) with a whole crew of people, including interns, residents, and medical students. I told them about the catheter threat and one guy spoke up. I don't remember his name or why he was there, but his words will always stay with me.

"When was the last time you wet the bed?" he asked politely.

"I don't know, probably ten years ago?" I said.

"Exactly," he replied, matter-of-factly. "You're not used to peeing when you're lying in bed. So get up, walk to the bathroom, and stand in front of the toilet. We want you to start walking around anyway, and I guarantee that it will work."

"Okay, you're the boss," I replied, hoping he was right.

After they all left, I hobbled to the bathroom. I stood in front of the toilet for what seemed like an eternity. The idea of getting a catheter was driving me crazy. I waited. I waited some more. I was growing convinced that I would never pee again. Ever.

Finally, the floodgates opened. I could feel the pressure lessen in my abdomen as the splashing sound in the toilet got louder and louder. It was maybe the best sound I could imagine hearing. My whole body was letting go of itself. It was the most glorious feeling ever. I felt such a sense of relief—for the obvious reason, and from knowing that I wouldn't need a catheter. I was already facing the miserable isolation radiation iodine treatments. Who needed a catheter on top of that?

For the first time in my life, peeing was a major accomplishment.

~Jasan Zimmerman, age 15

16

Chicken Soup for the Soul

Fighting Back

I was diagnosed with Stage II Hodgkin's Lymphoma in 1997 at age twenty-four.

I was lucky. I had a highly curable form of cancer, and it had been caught early. What made me even luckier, though, was that I lived in Buffalo, New York. Buffalo? When anybody thinks of Buffalo they imagine mounds and mounds of snow and the Bills and Lake Erie.

But the fact that I lived there made me lucky for one simple reason, and that is the Roswell Park Cancer Institute. "Roswell," as most people around here refer to it, was the nation's first comprehensive cancer center, and is still one of only forty in existence worldwide. When I was diagnosed, there wasn't a question in my mind about where I would go. With a facility like that in my backyard, why would I go anywhere else?

Thankfully, I was only in treatment for seven months, and was considered to be in remission by December of 1997. I only had one round of chemotherapy because of a horrifically painful allergic reaction, but I still lost my hair. I also endured twelve weeks of radiation treatments, which left me exhausted and sick to my stomach. My weight dropped from my pre-treatment high of 128 pounds to a low of 96.

The staff at Roswell really fought for me and that's what sticks with me the most, eleven years later.

One time, when I came in to have the usual blood work done, my oncologist, Dr. James Slack, didn't like the results. He also noticed that I was so weak I could barely sit up. After examining me, Dr. Slack wanted to admit me to the hospital. My insurance company was contacted but they refused to okay me for admittance.

From the other end of the clinic, as I lay in the exam room feeling so tired I could hardly stay awake, I heard Dr. Slack screaming at someone on the other end of the phone at the insurance company. They'd only seen the results of the blood work and hadn't seen me in person, so they said there wasn't enough reason, in their view, to admit me.

"Then, you come here and look at her; look at her good and then tell me she shouldn't be admitted!" Dr. Slack slammed down the phone. He calmed down after a few minutes and called them back, and I was admitted shortly thereafter. Dr. Slack typifies the kind of person who works at Roswell. Patients first.

Throughout my treatment, the entire staff—from the doctors and nurses to the tech staff and even the cafeteria workers and maintenance people—treated me with dignity and respect. It's such a positive, cheerful place, and I really got the sense that everyone was working toward a common goal. Roswell made me want to fight back and beat the cancer. Although I came to take this for granted, I also knew that, unfortunately, Roswell is not your typical hospital.

During the hours I spent in waiting rooms, I got to read a lot of magazines and brochures. One in particular caught my eye, an advertisement for The Ride For Roswell, a yearly bike-a-thon to raise money for research and patient care. My husband and I decided to bike in the next event, which would take place in late June of 1998. That year, I rode the shortest course available—nine miles—and was completely bushed by the end. I was so proud of myself for finishing the course, though!

All day long, other riders and volunteers made comments about something my husband and I had decided to do on the spur of the moment. We had taken white undershirts and wrote in plain black magic marker on each shirt, then tucked them into the back of our shorts so they could be seen from behind while we rode.

Mine said, "Roswell Park Saved My Life," while my husband's read, "Roswell Park Saved My Wife." A photographer even took a picture! Little did we know, but that picture would grace the cover of The Ride For Roswell brochure for the coming year!

My history with Roswell and The Ride For Roswell continues to this day. After all, what better way to fight back than to help plan the biggest fundraising event we have for more cancer research? Since I joined the committee I've served in various capacities and have also continued to ride. I'm proud of what I've accomplished personally, but what I'm most proud of is what The Ride itself has done for everyone else.

Each year, as I attend meeting after meeting and debate subjects as mundane as where to set up food tables and how many sound systems we need, I remember what it was like to be a cancer patient at Roswell. I think about the caring staff and about all the patients who have gone through their doors, some never to come out.

I think about the best moment of the entire day at The Ride, when the emcee asks the cancer survivors to raise their hands. As I raise my hand and watch scores of hands going up, I cry. Every single time.

I remember why I do whatever they ask of me every year, why I arrive at the crack of dawn to help set up, and why I go back to my friends, family, and colleagues every year to ask for donations. It's all so that other people don't have to go through what I did. I fight to fund research to rid the world of this dreadful disease.

I feel as if God let me survive so I could help other people fight too. I do it for the people I love, including my father, Richard, and my cousin, Debbie, who both survived cancer, and my aunt Yvonne and my friend Jeff, who didn't. I feel a responsibility to those who have fought and lived, and to those who have died. Roswell is doing something about that and I can't ignore the gift of life I was given when my cancer went into remission.

That's my way of fighting back.

~Amanda Racette

17

Chicken Soup
for the Soul

Positive

"Of course, you know it's cancer, so I want to tell you a couple of things."

I really didn't hear the rest of that sentence or the next few. All I heard was the word, "cancer." I didn't quite understand why the doctor used it. I felt okay, pretty good, actually, considering I'd just had surgery.

This whole odyssey came about because my annual physical had turned up some blood in my urine. My family physician referred me to a urologist. To be honest, I had noticed the color come and go over the past year, but I figured it was probably from too much booze on occasion or a couple of kidney punches. The urologist, Dr. Zaki, took an X-ray of my kidneys and the pictures showed enough stones to build a little house. Zaki, as he preferred to be called, with no title, decided he should check out my bladder.

There's only one way to get to the bladder without cutting, so he numbed me up and performed a cystourethroscopy. In this procedure, a tube with lights and lenses is inserted in the urethra and shoved into the bladder so the doctor can have a gander at the surrounding area.

Zaki tried to do this. There were so many stones clogging the channel, it was like trying to breech the Great Barrier Reef. Push and twist as he did, Zaki couldn't finesse the scope through. He was dumbfounded. He told me he'd never seen anything quite like this and that for the life of him, he couldn't understand how I was able to relieve myself.

I assured Zaki that I could, sometimes more than I'd like. As soon as I said that he did a small, knowing double take in my direction and let me know that he really wanted to check out my bladder. Right away! The only way to do that was to scrape the rockslide of stones out of the way so the scope could do its job. That meant surgery.

I phoned my wife. I was admitted, prepped, and put under.

I came to in a hospital bed, my wife sitting in a chair next to me. Zaki had been able to get the stones out of the way and let the scope into the bladder. He discovered a tumor, went to work scraping away at it but couldn't get it all because it had invaded the bladder wall. It was right around then that I heard him say that word. Cancer. He said it in an almost throwaway manner.

All I could say was, "Well, I guess it's my turn."

The next thing that occurred to me was, "Okay, how do I fight this thing?"

I didn't realize it then, but that gut reaction was one of the most effective and helpful things I could have done for myself. Time after time, physicians have seen that a positive attitude can help patients cope with disease-related problems and may tip the scales in their favor.

Considering that I've always been in pretty fair shape and I watch my diet, I wondered how I could have contracted bladder cancer in the first place. Zaki knew that I drank. After all, I work in nightclubs. Although he didn't pass judgment on me, he mentioned that I might want to tone that down a bit. He asked me if I smoked. Did I smoke? Holy cow! Only for about thirty-five years! Zaki said that I might have contracted cancer for a few different reasons but perhaps the biggest reason was the fact that I was a smoker. That threw me. I could understand lung cancer or throat cancer maybe, but bladder cancer?

I did some reading (actually my wife did) and she discovered Zaki was right. According to the American Cancer Society, "The greatest risk factor for bladder cancer is smoking. Smokers are more than twice as likely to get bladder cancer as nonsmokers." That was the day I became a nonsmoker.

Over the next eleven months, I was bombarded with very aggressive chemotherapy treatments because radiation was considered too risky in my case. I also underwent a very long and involved surgery, wherein I was pretty much split up the keel and had a fair amount of me removed, including my bladder.

I had all the usual side effects, including hair loss, nausea, and disorientation. One thing that did come and go, with considerable severity, was pain. Certainly there was pain from the surgery, recovering from an invasive procedure that entailed an incision the length of the Euphrates. There was also pain, varied and intense, that seemed to be part of the chemotherapy. I had pain medication in the hospital and a little bit when I returned home, but it was minimal and I did without as soon as possible. I chose to exclusively use imagery and visualization.

According to the American Society of Clinical Oncology, "Many imagery techniques are useful for pain and discomfort associated with treatment. You may benefit from simple visualization exercises in which you imagine a peaceful scene or a favorite memory or create a mental picture of a healing light that takes pain up and away."

My technique was different. Making my fight with cancer a little more personal and more in tune with my demeanor and background, I visualized a U.S. Army Ranger buddy of mine fighting the cancer in my system. Calling on my own military training, I fought alongside him, reminding myself of the old adage that pain is just fear leaving the body. Eventually, it worked.

All cancers are unique as are all treatments. My methods might not be right for anybody else, but they worked and are continuing to work for me. No matter how a person chooses to deal with cancer, the one constant has to be a positive, confident attitude.

In my case, that translates to a certain amount of prayer, together with a belligerent and aggressive posture toward the disease. Though a positive attitude on its own will not pull you through, it's a sure bet you will not pull through without it.

~Frank Emerson

18

Chicken Soup
for the Soul

The Change

t is called The Change — that time of life that leaves women forever altered. It can be life-affirming if a woman sails into and out of The Change at the appropriate age and under precise conditions.

I am advised that under perfect circumstances a woman will have a remarkable outcome and life forever after will be a sexually freeing, white-wearing, tea-on-the-veranda, garden-party-attending, blissful experience.

I have been told by some elder women compatriots that The Change is not as bad as it is portrayed to be. They tell me I will hardly notice, and they whisper to me about the dryness and how certain ointments fix that right up.

I have also heard that, along with The Change, a woman will inherit an enhanced form of wisdom and an unflappable strength. I have especially looked forward to this. Many of my post-menopausal women friends seem to have it all together. They seem so sure of themselves and I often envy their "take no crap" attitudes.

I am not going to take any crap! I am Woman! Hear me roar!

I am a different woman. At the age of forty, I am being dragged, kicking and screaming, into The Change. See for me, sailing was not an option. In order to fight a disease that could take my life, I've had to give up the parts of me that make me a woman. It's a form of female chemical castration. I feel this will not end well for me.

So far, I hate wearing white; it makes me look fat and I get dirty faster. I don't do garden parties. I have allergies. I have never been sexually inhibited and who the hell has the time to sit on a veranda all day sipping tea? Who even has a veranda? What are the other benefits? Where is that wisdom and bold new attitude? Oh, yes, and what about this memory loss problem I've developed that my doctor says is because I am not producing estrogen anymore. Was I told about that? Maybe I've just forgotten.

And about that dryness, a minor blip on the menopause radar, compared to the night sweats and the hot flashes. Since the beginning of time, women have come up with these cute acronyms and polite phrases to describe the side effects of The Change. I find not one thing cute about sitting next to an industrial fan, trying to cool off when it's forty-eight degrees in the building.

"My own personal summer" or "my senior moment" is not fanciful or whimsical when you have just sweated through your new silk blouse in a meeting with beautiful women in their mid- to late-twenties with names like Amber or Skye who don't have a clue about why I have to excuse myself every fifteen minutes to get some air.

Hell, I'm burning up!

But it's not their fault. I hope they will sail into The Change.

I do admit that I have become a bit wiser and stronger and yes, I take no crap! But I cannot rightly attribute it all to The Change. I owe a large part of it to my own experience with a disease that has taught me to value life and that is teaching me that life is to be lived out loud. I am stronger because having or showing weakness is not conducive to a full and complete recovery. I am wiser because I have figured out a ton of creative ways to motivate myself to get up and go to work every day.

Most days I want to stay home in bed and watch CNN all day. I have become adept at answering questions about my cancer experience without crying and with a truthfulness that doesn't scare the hell out of people. Even more significantly, when my meal is served incorrectly, I will send it back. Life is too short to eat an under-cooked steak that's over-priced.

The Change has surely changed me.

~Za Zette Scott

19

Deal With It

noticed a lump on my neck while shaving and thought it was a cyst which could simply be removed in my doctor's office. I was overwhelmed when it turned out to be head and neck cancer.

When bad things happen to me, my typical first reaction is to seek blame so that my anger can be appropriately directed. Cancer doesn't allow that. At first, I thought the cause of my cancer might have been secondary smoke from my mother, who always had a lit cigarette nearby, or maybe it was from my grandfather's dry cleaning business and the carcinogenic chemicals I was exposed to while I worked there for seven years through high school and college.

Thankfully, I realized right away that the two people I admired most but who also may have exposed me to cancer would have just said, "Cancer? Tough cookies. Get over it and move on." And, they would have been right. It didn't matter how or why.

For me, cancer quickly became more about looking forward and dealing head on with what was to come. Eventually, through reflection and research, I realized that how I got cancer meant little compared to how I would deal with it.

Like many people in a similar circumstance, I scanned the Internet for every piece of information I could find and did a fair amount of number crunching. The bottom line looked like only one-third of those diagnosed survived past five years. Not great news for a forty-year-old with a wife, five-year-old twins (boy and girl), and a load of bills to pay in the future. It turns out I was lucky that it was discovered early and that I ended up being treated at Memorial Sloan-Kettering Cancer Center, whose statistics I later learned are significantly better than what the Internet presents.

I was told I would have a chunk—one muscle, a vein, and sixty-one lymph nodes—of my neck removed and my left arm would lose fifty percent of its mobility. There would be no guarantees, of course, but theoretically, at least, I would live.

Because my kids were so young, I wanted to do everything I could to fight the cancer, win or lose. If my children only remembered me for not giving up, it would have been enough. The thought of looking back and not knowing that I had done everything I could was potentially the scariest outcome I could imagine. That made it easier for me to take the more aggressive of two proposed approaches with my cancer treatment. Anything less than that wouldn't have been trying as hard as I could. So, when the choice came down to removing the tumor and waiting, or a half neck dissection followed by radiation and chemo, the decision was relatively easy.

With that in mind, I had to find the best overall approach as fast as I could. Some people need a lot of support and others don't. For better or for worse, I've always dealt with tough situations on my own. I had been a long-distance runner and although it was rewarding, I would have preferred something less painful and lonely. However, since cancer is both painful and lonely, I had a pretty good understanding that at the end of the road I would probably throw up and feel sore but eventually also gain a sense of accomplishment and the satisfaction that I had pushed as hard as I could and succeeded.

My treatment included two surgeries, seven weeks of radiation, and a few all-day rounds of chemo—as my son said, "not fun." I couldn't sleep lying down for six months. I went though narcotic withdrawal when I rushed to get off the medicine and back to work. My weight dropped from 180 pounds to 115 at its lowest point.

Only my wife and a few people from work were aware of what was going on until six weeks after the radiation stopped. I didn't even tell my brothers or my parents. With young kids at home requiring and deserving full attention, the last thing I wanted was the consistent reminder to my wife from daily phone calls checking on how I was doing. I wasn't doing well! And I didn't have any desire to keep repeating that fact to anyone.

My wife realized the need to give me space to block out any noise from well-intentioned family and friends, thereby allowing me to focus on coping with the treatment. Controlling what I could and trusting others with what I couldn't was the toughest part for me. I moved into a separate room for four months to deal with radiation, chemo, night sweats, and generally not sleeping through the night. This also allowed my wife to sleep and make things as normal as possible for our kids. No daily phone calls or visits from family or friends required my wife to repeat the same crappy story over and over again.

The best thing I have ever done is to marry a woman who is very strong and didn't reach out for her own support group, which would have been her right. She respected my privacy and had the same positive attitude I had about attacking the situation as a team in our own individual ways. A strong partner is critical for anyone who chooses this approach.

Our kids know I was sick but now, at age nine, they don't recall or worry much about it. But all along, they were my motivation. I thought every day about all the things I would want to tell them as they progressed from kindergarten to marriage. Realizing I might not be there to scold or motivate them forced me to think about what I would like to say to them as they grew up. I put together a list a things that would likely come up each year of their lives and how I would suggest they handle it. People have to make their own choices in life and when mistakes are made they need to make the most out of that situation as well. I figured that what I wanted to tell them at age sixteen should probably be said at fourteen. Hopefully, I'll now have the chance to tell them, myself.

I ended treatment three years ago and now get checked about three times a year. While I have one hundred percent movement, I still have a permanently stiff neck with some chronic pain, which to me is a fantastic outcome. Cancer will always be a part of my past but although I look at life differently since getting through it, I try hard not to make it something I think about on a daily basis. I care less now about what most people think, and care more about what my wife and kids think. I am not religious, but I do believe in God—a Higher Being. The tests I've been given have made my life more fulfilling, and ultimately I think I'm a better husband, friend, and father.

~Robert Gelnaw

20

Moments

"Yes, it's confirmed. It's alveolar rhabdomyosarcoma, although your son is a little old to have this particular childhood cancer."

"What? Nick? He's only eighteen! He graduates from high school next month. Are you sure?"

"Yes, it's Stage IV."

The words took a few seconds to register. I tried listening to the procedures that needed to be done before hospital admission.

"He only has a ten percent chance of survival."

How would I gather myself before seeing Nick?

Alveolar rhabdomyosarcoma, adriamycin, ifosfamide, mesna, maxillectomy, resection, viable cells, radiation, tumor board, neutropenic, Hickman port, transfusions, bone marrow, biopsy, malignancy—all of these presented monumental moments of confusion.

During Nick's very first day of his first round of chemo, a very wise nurse told me, "Our doctors and nurses are excellent. The hospital is excellent. However, he's your son and your responsibility, so always know what is going on. Ask questions. Get copies of everything. Research the drugs. Keep notes on what meds work or don't. I'll help you learn what to be concerned with on the lab results." She made a difference in helping me regain moments of clarity and confidence.

My two best girlfriends (there with me when Nick was born)

came in to the hospital, singing, "You Are My Sunshine," dressed from head to toe as fairy godmothers, including wands. This was their first visit during Nick's first, week-long round of chemo. Subsequent visits included cowboys, pirates, clowns, Groucho Marx doctors, penguins, and giant grapes. They always brought armfuls of treats, presents, and laughter. These moments of true friendship are invaluable and Nick and I cherish them. Nick has received many spiritual blessings, as well. Our church dedicated an entire day of fasting for him and hundreds of our youth carried on the fast through the evening. He has received a prayer shawl and quilt. Several denominations have included him in their church prayers. Many are people we know; thousands are not.

The strongest demonstration of the power of prayer came during one of Nick's most difficult nights. With severe sores in his mouth, throat, and nose he was on a feeding tube. My 6'3" son weighed only 125 pounds. He was home, on the couch, too weak to go to his own bed. He slept with his prayer quilt and shawl wrapped around him.

As I checked on him, he woke up and whispered, "Mom, would you pray with me?" For the first time in many years, he let me hold him in my arms. We were blessed with the amazing relationship a mother and son can have and the comfort that God is with us and everything would be okay.

I also have two daughters, ages sixteen and eleven, living at home. Both are avid softball players on competitive traveling teams. One beautiful fall night, Nick was fresh out of the hospital, on a feeding tube and very weak. But he felt like sitting in the ballpark with blankets and recliners in the grass. He embraced the opportunity to enjoy the atmosphere under a full harvest moon with the smell of hamburgers and fries and the spectacular view of the Wasatch Mountains as a backdrop to the ballfields.

It was a moment of being back to normal, full of serenity for all of our family.

More than anything, I cherish the people who have made it possible for me to survive:

The nurse who brings me a chilled Diet Coke at 7:30 A.M. after a long night in the hospital, without asking.

Our local hockey team, which donated 100% of one games ticket sales to the Huntsman Cancer Institute, and introduced Nick to the team.

The get-well letter and lei Nick received from a three-year-old girl in Hawaii.

Nick's friends visiting him in the hospital to play rambunctious games of dice until well past midnight.

Neighbors offering to let our daughters spend the night whenever there's an emergency.

All of these people have provided beautiful moments of kindness.

And they co-exist with moments of staff meetings, laundry, e-mail, grocery shopping, birthday parties, softball practice, conference calls, church, haircuts, house guests, music recitals, parent-teacher conferences, hockey games, paying bills, watering plants, feeding dogs, fixing dinner, tennis tournaments, primping for proms, attending funerals, cleaning house, changing the oil, snow blowing, braiding hair....

But all are temporary.

What remains is all that I've learned from this experience. The sorrow and pain are fleeting, if I consciously envision myself letting go once the moment has passed. Another moment always awaits and it may be full of hope or peace, ready to replace the difficult one I've just released.

When it was time for Nick to graduate, his white blood count was barely high enough for him to even attend. As his name was read, "Nicholas William Raitt, Magna Cum Laude," his graduating class stood up with stunningly loud applause. Tears of gratitude filled my moment of pride. Nick seemed to float a full foot off the ground for the rest of the day.

Not long after, while finishing dinner one night, our older daughter asked if we had any index cards at home for her homework. No, I replied. She asked if we would go get some for her. No again.

When we reminded her she could drive herself the whole three-quarters of a mile to the store, she lamented, "But look at me! My hair is a mess, I have on sweats and no makeup. You never know who I may run into."

She went on until Nick finally said, "Carly! I have one eyebrow! No hair! No eyelashes! I've been to the store twice today!"

In a moment of perfect perspective, she smiled, put on her shoes and went to the store.

Moments like this have made all of us stronger, through the power of gratitude, a stronger faith in God, a stronger stomach, a stronger appreciation of time, and a stronger ability to love my husband, my children, and my friends.

~Lori Brower

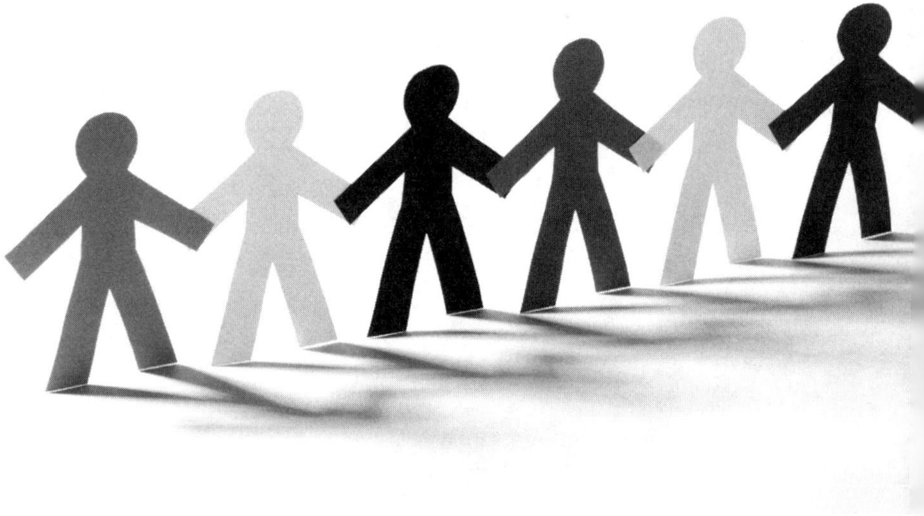

The Cancer Book

For Better and For Worse

When you come to the end of your rope, tie a knot and hang on.

~*Franklin D. Roosevelt*

21

Glad to Be Alive

My body feels foreign to me, as if I'm an alien inhabiting the shell of another species. I rise from bed with difficulty and clumsily shuffle to the wheelchair. My spirit flits freely from one delighted thought to the next, like a butterfly, visiting flower after flower.

I'm going home!

I remember the flurry of excitement when I discovered I could wiggle the big toe on my right foot the morning after a surgeon removed the tumor from my spine. Before the operation, I hadn't been able to move anything below my armpits. The tears in my doctor's eyes had seemed so odd to me. Why would anyone cry over a wiggling toe?

The nurse wheels me down the hallway. If I had the energy, I'd run from this place. But I must be content to roll along at my escort's pace. In the elevator, we descend in silence.

My mom is fetching my car, which will hopefully be easy to get into.

"There she is!" I eagerly tell the nurse.

"Careful, honey," the nurse murmurs, as she grabs my arm to steady me. With some effort, I land successfully in the seat next to my mom, and the nurse helps me wrangle my legs inside.

"Thank you," I reply, glad to be free of her care.

"How are you?" my mom asks.

"I wonder if I truly believed I'd ever return home again."

I thought of that first time I was forced out of bed after the surgery.

"We're going to work on getting you up today," the nurse had said. She'd strapped a belt around my hips and kept a tight rein on it to keep me from wobbling uncontrollably. I raised one leg and set it down a few inches in front of me, tightening my grip on her hand as I battled gravity.

"When you walk, your heels need to hit the ground first," she instructed. "You walk heel-toe, heel-toe." I couldn't take a single step on my own.

Now, I'm so relieved to see something other than the pastel walls of the hospital in which I'd been trapped for so long. I feast my eyes on our surroundings as we ride in happy silence. I treasure each sight, from the soaring overpass of the expressway to the pipe-studded mounds of the garbage dump. My body feels lighter as we near home. Here comes my exit, my post office, my street, and finally, my house. Each one is a deep pleasure to see.

"We haven't installed a railing yet, so you'll have to hold onto me," my mom reports.

This pleases me. I want everything to be just the way it was.

"Maybe you won't have to," I say hopefully, willing the doctors to be wrong about my bleak prognosis for future mobility.

My mom helps me stand, walk, and climb the steps. My first stop is the bathroom.

"I can flush!" I proclaim triumphantly. No more counting every drop. Even this small change brings me untold satisfaction.

My mother smiles, appreciating this small victory nearly as much as I do. She takes my arm and steadies me as I shuffle to the couch.

"I don't want you to leave this couch without me," she sternly admonishes. "I don't want you falling and hurting yourself."

"I don't think I'm going anywhere too soon," I reply, sinking into the cushions, exhausted. I was eighteen years old but I didn't mind my mother's admonishment.

For the next year, the routine would be the same. Every three weeks, I would be driven to the hospital, where I patiently waited to be admitted, to be hydrated, and to receive my chemo treatments. After the better part of a week filled with restless channel surfing, fitful round-the-clock naps, shuffling walks down hallways that smelled of antiseptic and echoed with beeps and human groans, I became free again.

For a day or two, I would feel good. But inevitably, infection set in and after another day or two at home battling an aching throat and a rising fever, I would once again be admitted to the hospital. The IV antibiotics killed the infection, and eventually, I would head home. That left me about a week to huddle in bed or on the couch, gathering strength for the next round of chemo.

Some day it would all come to an end. My final treatment would be complete, and this time, I would be staying here for good.

But for now, I inhale deeply, remembering the scent of home. The curtains, the television, the computer desk—all are right where I left them, reassuring me that not everything in life has changed. I close my eyes, feeling the warmth of the sunshine through the window. The sun has never felt so friendly; the couch has never felt so soft, and I have never been so glad to be alive.

• • •

That was me, back when Ewings Sarcoma, primarily a cancer of the bone and connective tissue, had taken over my life. Doctors reassured me of my progress toward remission. Family and friends surrounded me with encouragement. Scheduling activities depended upon my chemo routine and level of fatigue. When all of that ended, after I was finally able to walk again, after I had surprised my neurosurgeon by learning to run and eventually even ski, I was expected to return to "life as usual."

But my mind could not recover at the same rate as my body. The doctors labeled it post traumatic stress disorder; I thought of it as a collection of frustrating fears that made my life difficult. I cried when plans changed, unable to adjust. I cried when family members went away for an evening, afraid they might not return. I was afraid to go out on my own, even for a quick trip to the store or a meeting with friends.

It's been six years since I finished chemo. Externally I appear fine, but internally I still struggle. While everyone assumes that my life is normal, I know that it's not. Those who meet me have no way of knowing my history, no way of knowing that who I am is not who I might have been. I still cry when plans change. I let my family go about their daily business, but long trips away still make me nervous. I go places alone, but nowhere unfamiliar.

I will never be the same. Counseling helps but I don't want to merely cope. I want to live without the baggage.

My experience with cancer is both a badge of honor and a thorn in my side. I am proud to be a survivor but I will always wonder what might have been.

~Shereen D. Vinke

22

Chicken Soup
of the Soul

One Ball, Two Strikes

My story begins nine years ago. At thirty-one years old, I was the cardiovascular director for one of the world's largest pharmaceutical companies. I was married to my college girlfriend, expecting our first child.

I had a Masters in reproductive endocrinology and a PhD in biochemistry. I published papers on detoxification proteins in testicular tissue. When my right testicle was getting larger, I knew what it likely meant.

I secured an urgent appointment with a young urologist. I'll call him "Dr. A." I told him about my symptoms.

"My right testis has gotten larger and it is not thermoregulating correctly." In other words, it's not going up and down like it should when the temperature changes.

Dr. A ordered an ultrasound and other tests. He began buzzing around my privates. I saw dark and light areas on the screen. He buzzed around the side that I thought was normal. The left didn't look like the right.

"See this area? That's problematic. Please get dressed. We'll talk in my office."

I went into Dr. A's office. "You have testicular cancer. I can get you in for surgery in eight days."

All I heard was that I would have an eight-day wait to get a cancer out of my body. I told him to book it. I guess he was surprised that I didn't just fall apart on him. I needed to be alive for my wife and kid. Losing one testicle didn't worry me too much.

I called my wife and asked her to come home from work. My mother, a retired nurse, was able to get me in to see the chief of the urology department at the university hospital. I'll call him "Dr. B." I didn't think I needed another opinion as I thought Dr A's was solid.

Dr. B was in his sixties. There were dozens of certificates on his walls. I told him my symptoms. With a latex glove on his hand, he manipulated the testis that I thought was cancerous. The whole process took five seconds.

"You have a tumor and it has to come out. I can get you into surgery tomorrow."

I decided that Dr. B was my man. I thought about how the new generation of physicians was being trained. Dr. B laid his hands on me and made the same call as Dr. A had with all of his technology. If machines drive diagnoses, what kind of physicians are we training?

Dr. B discussed with me the various types of testicular cancers, the staging of the tumor, and options for treatment. We scheduled my surgery.

I went home. I called my brothers and a few of my best friends to tell them what was going on. It got harder each time because it hit me that I was talking about me.

My extended family joined me at the hospital on that Saturday morning. The admitting nurse told me that I was to go home that afternoon. I didn't like the idea of going home that day. I was about to have my lower right abdomen opened, my testicle pushed up, out, and snipped away. I felt that I deserved an overnight.

In the operating room, I spoke with Dr. B as he marked me up with a pen to indicate which was the part that had to go. He told me that he might be able to identify the tumor type during surgery and would inform me when I awoke.

I woke up in my hospital room. Everyone from the morning was there. I felt awful. The incision area hurt. I knew that when the meds wore off, it was going to suck. A nurse came in to tell me that she wanted me to walk.

"You're joking!" I thought.

I never shied away from pain. I had spent four of my college summers doing swimming pool repair and renovation, bleeding every day. At the time of my surgery, I was playing in a baseball league, getting spiked and hit by pitches. It wasn't the pain I was afraid of. The problem was that I felt disoriented and nauseous. I wasn't ready. As a trained biochemist and medical school instructor, the fact that I knew more about physiology didn't have any pull in the practice of medicine.

The nurse made me stand.

As I did, my blood pressure dropped and I became nauseous. We had discovered in the operating room that I had needed additional anesthesia. However, no one had told the recovery nurse to take it easy on me for a few more hours. So, I had to find a place to vomit. Vomiting is awful when you have a five-inch incision on your lower abdomen.

I was allowed to stay until 2:00 P.M. the same day. I felt like an unwanted guest. "Okay, we cut you open and took your nut. Party's over, go home."

Since I had great insurance, I went to a prestigious cancer center for follow-up. I learned that once you are a cancer patient with good insurance, you become clinically indicated for every treatment even if you don't need it. Upon consultation, I was told that they wanted to start my outpatient treatments by doing a lymph angiogram. In this procedure, an incision was to be cut into my foot and dye pumped into my lymphatic system. My surgical pathology said that it was unlikely that the cancer spread, and therefore there was little reason to check my entire lymph system. As an educated medical researcher, I realized that I was a way for others to make money.

"Here is a cancer guy; we can do things to him."

I didn't need that procedure. I said no way. It concerned me that there are cancer patients who are not informed enough to say "no" to certain procedures.

I met with a radiologist a few weeks later. We discussed my options. If I didn't get radiation, I'd have an 80% chance of a five-year survival. If I did get radiation, I'd increase that to 95%. With all of the knowledge I had, the right thing to do was just watch and wait. One thing about cancer though, no matter how much you know, it all goes out the window when it is you and your family. Radiation wasn't easy and there could be consequences, such as secondary tumors. The additional 15% survival seemed worth the risk. A decision I would later regret.

My radiologist recommended that I bank sperm if I wanted more children, as the radiation could damage my healthy testicle. I declined. I was exhausted from seeing white coats.

I learned a new cancer patient humiliation. In order to protect my healthy testicle from collateral radiation, my genitals were encased in a heavy lead clamshell ball contraption. It was always cold. A female nurse always clamped it on.

Radiation itself was easy to receive. The side effects were lousy. I would suffer from exhaustion or bouts of vomiting. I lost some hair. Eventually I developed radiation colitis, something I would battle fiercely and desperately for the next five years. I should have taken the watch-and-wait path.

Six months after the initial diagnosis, my son was born. A little more than three years later, my miracle daughter was born.

I was declared cancer-free after five years of follow-up. What I learned will stay with me forever. Under times of great stress, the health care system has a tendency to push toward what is protocol. In fact, it is during those times that we need most to be treated as individuals.

~Jonathan Rowe

23

My Mantra

February 2005.

I am okay, I remind myself.

I'm lying on a stretcher, headed for an operating room in the same hospital where I work five shifts a week. I'm a registered nurse. I know a lot of the doctors by name. I could walk this campus blindfolded. But I've never been here as a patient.

It feels cold in this waiting area. I don't know if it's from the cold or from nerves. I close my eyes, thinking. I'm here for brain surgery. Someone I've met for fifteen minutes is going to slice open my skull and remove a tumor from the right frontal lobe of my brain.

At this moment, I am not thinking of dying. I am thinking of how weird it feels to know that someone, other than God, is going to see such an intimate, vital part of me. It's my brain, for crying out loud. This guy, this surgeon, is going to touch it with his hands. I can't get that out of my head. I shiver all over again.

A young guy in blue scrubs walks up, smiling, and hands me a purple Sharpie. He points to my head.

"Make an 'X' where your tumor is," he explains. I'm starting to feel a little groggy.

"You're kidding," I say, looking up at him and grinning. It's a normal magic marker. "For something like brain surgery, you'd think they'd be a little more high tech."

He chuckles. "Yep, that's what you'd think."

After I mark a clumsy "X" on the upper right side of my forehead, he rolls me to the operating area.

"You're gonna be just fine," he says.

I nod. I hope he's right.

Nine hours later, I open my eyes. I feel like a million tiny ants are crawling all over me. I itch everywhere. I scratch fiercely. A week from now, I'll be covered with tiny, open sores from what I discover is the morphine. I'll need it for the pain, but it will wreck my body. I'm in so much pain I can barely keep my eyes open. Everything hurts. It's like the world's greatest migraine. Light cuts like a knife. My mother's soft voice sounds like the shrill scream of a train.

But I am awake.

I am alive.

I repeat that thought over and over. It becomes my mantra when the pain gets too deep.

I am alive. I am alive. I am alive.

• • •

February 2006.

I have passed the one-year mark. My tumor was not benign and the doctor said there was an eighty percent chance of it returning within three years. He congratulated me on surviving and recommended radiotherapy, and if it came back, chemo. He said I should make out a will, just in case.

He was an excellent surgeon, but he didn't know how devastating the whole ordeal would become for me. He was not a psychiatrist. He took out the tumor. He healed me physically. He didn't intend to hold my hand for the rest of my life. He didn't say a word about the Frontal Lobe Syndrome I would face, the mounting confusion and mental fogging that would force me out of work for two long years.

I am not who I was before the surgery. I was optimistic and carefree. I ran on the beach with my kids and my dogs.

I haven't properly recognized my own children for six months. I know they are mine, but I don't know which daughter goes with which name, or which one is oldest.

I can't remember the words for ordinary things. Making a salad, I ask someone to hand me "the green ball in the refrigerator." Crossing the street, I cling tightly to my daughter's hand.

"Do you go on green?" I ask in a panic, "or red?"

I've become a hypochondriac. Every symptom drives me to the doctor.

I tell my wonderful new husband, Dave, that I hope we live together for a long time, "but you never know." I try to enjoy life, but there's always a cloud hanging over me. I won't relax for two more years, at least. I look for the three-year mark in 2008.

"Everything will be great in 2008," has become my new mantra.

•••

February 2007.

As I edge closer to my target, I have become easier to live with but now I am fat. Now, I eat chocolate, lots of it, and pasta, and bread. Food comforts me. When I was a little girl, every time I was sad, or scared, or hurting, my mother offered me food. We didn't have a medicine cabinet filled with pills. We had chicken soup, fresh-squeezed orange juice, and loads of sweets.

I am beginning to believe that I will live a normal life. Seven MRIs have been clean. No more tumors. I stopped the Dilantin this year. I had an entire year free from seizures. I can drive again. The doctor who treats me for Frontal Lobe Syndrome tells me "it can go either way." I can stay on disability or try working again. My neurological testing shows some delay, but it's improving. I am remembering more.

But I look in the mirror and don't recognize the woman looking back. Still, something good is happening. I am getting in touch with my faith. I talk to God openly. I ask Him why I had the tumor. I thank Him for letting me live.

• • •

June 2008.

My life has come full circle. My daughters, Zoe, Chloe, and Caroline, are beautiful and full of life. I will start work again, as a nurse at my younger girls' elementary school.

I've gone three whole months without thinking about tumors, or cancer, or chemo, or dying. I am healthy and whole. I am okay, I say to myself, over and over. I am okay.

It has become my mantra.

~Donna Reames Rich

24

Survivors Rule!

D ecember 27th, 1995.

I was twenty-one years old and one semester away from graduating from college, en route to film school with musical ambitions to become the next John Williams. I'd been classically trained for more than ten years with a romp through jazz, new age, electronic, and pop/rock. I wanted nothing more than to be creative and write music for film and TV.

But first, someone had to explain why my speech was slurring, why I kept fainting, why I had crippling headaches, and, most importantly, why my left hand, my dominant one, had lost all of its fine motor coordination, rendering me unable to sit at the piano and play, grip a pen, or type on the computer.

I had an MRI and the next six months were a blur. It went something like this: scan, brain tumor, surgery, cancer diagnosis, lots of radiation therapy. And all I wanted to do that entire time was graduate in May and play the piano. I wanted to forget that cancer had ever happened.

That was thirteen years ago and, considering I was given a fifty percent chance of living for five years, I think I can safely say it's been fun proving my prognosticators wrong, although I do remember them saying my hair would grow back.

It took me five years to regain full use of my left hand and play piano again, so instead of heading off to film school I spent several years building a new life, working in IT, marketing, and advertising. I grew far away from cancer and everything and everyone surrounding it.

The release of my first solo piano album (which was written in my head all the years I was assiduously retraining myself), unexpectedly hurled me back into the cancer world I was so excited to have finally escaped from. I had made the album to regain what cancer had taken away from me. Invariably, what got the most attention was the story of how I had finally overcome the effects of cancer. The response was unanticipated and I became a spokesman for many others who shared a common experience.

And I've never looked back.

I quit my cushy job on Madison Avenue. More than 200 concert appearances and speaking engagements later, I've given in to destiny by reinvesting myself—mind, body, and spirit—into the world of cancer advocacy.

The bottom line is, no one should have to go through what I went through, but if they do, they should not feel like they're the only one on the planet. Isolation is the number one psychosocial issue facing cancer survivors between the ages of fifteen and thirty-nine, a population referred to as young adult. I took up the cause of young adult cancer advocacy because little had been done to recognize this oft-forgotten community within the cancer continuum.

Roughly 68,000 young adults are stricken with cancer each year, up two hundred percent over the past twenty years. But survival rates for young adults remain largely unchanged. Rhetorically, if I were diagnosed again today with the same cancer, my outcome would be the same, in spite of all the major advances in prevention, early detection, and medical technology.

In 2007, I founded the I'm Too Young For This! Cancer Foundation, a nonprofit organization that advocates on behalf of young adults affected by cancer. As a national voice for the next generation of survivors, we have become a global support community.

One month after our launch, we were profiled in *The New York Times* and soon after, we were ranked one of *Time's* Best 50 Websites for 2007. I was invited to join the Google Health Advisory Council to represent the interests of the more than one million young adult survivors in the United States.

Thanks to a new relationship with Lifetime Television, millions of viewers watched as I guest-starred on an episode of *Side Order of Life* as the host of a hip cancer support "happy hour" where one of the show's main characters (a survivor herself) goes to hang out with likeminded peers. It was the first time in television history where a young adult was accurately represented—not as a bald and pitied victim but as a "normal" person. It was a wake up call for Johnny Couch Potato and showed what young adults with cancer look like.

There are currently few clinical trials or cancer research projects focused on young adults. Why? We're too small a population, I guess. The young adult cancer problem is only going to be solved by and within the young adult community, from the demographic that's brought us MySpace, Facebook and YouTube.

It's my personal mission not only to mobilize and activate GenX/Y but to develop our own "me generation" philanthropy model to solve our own problems with the same fervor we've shown for *American Idol*. We can create lasting social change to overcome this generational health disparity. We fight because remission is not a cure and survivorship is all the rage.

Thirteen years have passed since I was initially diagnosed. I'm now married, fertile (again), an author, a radio show host, a blogger, and big mouth rabble-rouser in the cancer universe. I couldn't ask for a better life and I have cancer to thank for it. I know it sounds weird but here we are, and I wouldn't rather be anywhere else.

~Matthew Zachary

25

Stronger

T wo frogs fell down a well. A group of frogs gathered to watch, and they yelled down at the frogs, "You'll never get back up!" One of the frogs became discouraged and gave up and drowned. The other frog kept jumping and eventually got out of the well. The frogs that had been watching asked, "Why did you keep trying when we told you you'd never make it?" The frog replied, "Oh, I thought they were words of encouragement!"

My mom told me that story after the doctors determined that I had osteosarcoma. Finally, a month into my freshman year at college, I knew why I had been limping the past five months. There was a cancerous tumor in my left femur. After a month of scans, tests, and chemo, I underwent an operation to remove my knee and parts of my femur and tibia and had them replaced with a titanium prosthesis. Six months of chemo followed, along with a regimen of physical therapy that I had to endure if I ever wanted to walk again.

I thought, if Mom is willing to tell me stories about talking amphibians, there must be a good moral. She also said, "You don't have to win every battle to win the war." Over the next nine months, I had to learn not to resign myself to the fate predicted by some of my doctors. I struggled with everything—uncertainty about the future, hair loss, nausea, fear of needles, weekly blood tests, ER visits, major operations, a biopsy where they didn't give me enough local anesthetic, lack of sleep, mouth sores, trouble and pain with walking and bending my leg, and being stared at in public—and I'm glad I did.

The whole ordeal has given me more confidence in my ability to defy expectations, as well as a deep appreciation for what my family and friends will do for me. What doesn't kill you really does make you stronger, and though at first I thought everything would kill me, I now have a new appreciation for a lot of things.

I'm also having more fun at the hospital and spending less time in bed. When I arrived for my most recent session, I announced a crutch decorating party in the playroom. Six hours later, after playing games and talking, we all got tired and retired to our rooms.

I ran into two of my doctors.

"Natalie, you're like the poster-child for chemotherapy. Do you have any idea how hard I try to get these kids out of bed? And then you come along and everyone's in the playroom."

I said, "Well, maybe they just got really bored."

Then she replied, "Nope, pretty sure it's just you."

So that was nice to hear. Natalie, the optimistic frog!

A team of six doctors tours the hospital each day, spending a few minutes with every patient. This is my favorite part of the day and amuses me to no end. Personally, I don't find my mouth sores very interesting, but the doctors are fascinated. They gather in a semi-circle around my bed, one of them shines a light in my mouth, and they all simultaneously lean forward as far as they can and crane their necks to see, and let out a collective "Ooooh."

The next day I decided to treat them to something really fascinating—my leg! I rolled up my pants and demonstrated my leg-bending skills. They asked a bunch of questions about skin sensitivity, etc., and then did the whole leaning in to look at my mouth routine again.

They make me feel like a celebrity. Only, instead of walking the red carpet, I'm sitting in a blue hospital bed, and instead of flash bulbs going off in my face, they're shining lights in my eyes to see if my pupils dilate, and instead of wearing a gown designed by someone famous, I am wearing a hospital gown that is a little too breezy in the back, if you get my draft, er, drift.

I am getting stronger every day, physically and mentally. I no longer get winded walking to the kitchen in the morning. I don't get tired from standing up long enough to make a sandwich. I go out of the house almost every day, be it to physical therapy, lunch, or both, and I don't need a break just from walking to the car. I am also better at getting up from the floor or a chair, and just moving in general. My sister even says I'm "stealthy." While I wouldn't quite call myself that (you can hear me coming because I use a cane, just in case), I feel so much better.

My anxiety has lessened. I have people praying for me who I don't even know, in places I've never been. With so much support from well-wishers, I can't help but be cheerful.

When I went to get fitted for my leg brace, I was dutifully wearing my protective mask, something I hated to wear in public not so long ago. The lady who was doing the fitting asked me, "How did you break your femur?" and I realized she didn't consider me a convalescing weirdo wearing a mask, but rather just a normal person who broke a bone. I was even more surprised to find myself glibly replying, "Oh, I didn't break it, I just have cancer."

The other day, I went out with my boyfriend for dinner. Someone sneezed, so I busted out my trusty mask. A little girl, still too young to understand the concept of speaking in hushed tones, immediately turned to her mom and, while pointing at me, loudly asked (twice), "Mommy, why is that girl wearing a mask?"

About a month ago, this would have been my cue to turn away abruptly, tears spilling from my eyes, complaining bitterly about "looking like a freak," but I found myself unperturbed. I turned to the girl, smiled and said something like, "I have to wear a mask because there are germs in the air and that makes it easy for me to get sick."

The girl said "Oh!" and proceeded to ask me if I wanted to hear her sing "The Bunny Song." I used to glare right back at kids staring at me (I knew they didn't know any better but I felt like a walking freak show), but now I realize that, like Mom told me, once you tell kids, they don't really care, much less think you're a freak. They also really understand stories about drowning frogs.

I have made major strides. I've accepted the fact that I am currently a cancer patient, but that's not going to prevent me from going out and enjoying myself. I no longer think that every person who looks at me because I'm wearing a mask and have no hair is judging me. I even took off my hat at the restaurant, something I used to be ashamed to do, even at home! I finally realized that other people weren't judging me right about the same time that I finally stopped judging myself.

~Natalie Flechsig, age 19

26

Chicken Soup for the Soul

Marry Me

The first time they found cancer was in 2004, when Victoria was eight-and-a-half months pregnant with our daughter and felt a mass under her left breast. The doctor delivered Amira, and a week later Victoria had a biopsy. We sat in the surgeon's office and I held her hand when he delivered the news.

"Victoria, you have Stage IIIb invasive ductal carcinoma, a fast-growing cancer."

I wanted to scream. How could she have cancer? She was only thirty-four years old. She had just had a baby!

On the ride home, Victoria whispered, "Charles, where did this come from? I have no family history of breast cancer. How am I going to tell the boys? Am I going to die and leave them without a mother?"

At home, she huddled under the covers. Her mom and sister came. The days wore on.

"Honey," I begged one morning. "Get up. We have to tell the boys."

"I can't, Charles."

"They need to know," I persisted. Victoria shared a powerful bond with her two teenaged sons from a previous marriage.

She forced herself out of bed. We called Adam and Adrien into the dining room. She struggled to say the words.

A week later, Victoria had a mastectomy. Back home, she was

filled with sorrow at the loss of her breast, but to me, that was only a small, physical part of her.

"Marry me, Victoria," I blurted out one night. We'd been together more than three years and had discussed marriage before.

"Charles, how could you still want me? I'm sick. Why saddle yourself with a wife who could die?"

"I love you and want to marry you." I held her until she fell asleep in my arms, her tears drying on my shirt.

Victoria endured radiation and then chemo, but when her gorgeous, long hair began falling out in clumps, she crumbled. She wore scarves and wigs, but to me, she was always lovely.

A few months after her mastectomy, a colleague invited her to run in the Susan G. Komen Race for the Cure in Orange County.

"I'm going to do it," Victoria said. "There are women there who are two-, three-, even four-time survivors. If they can do it, I can too!" A warm smile spread across her cheeks.

A year after her first bout with cancer, Victoria was pregnant again. We'd been told there was no chance of conceiving. This child would be a miracle. But the doctors advised us to terminate the pregnancy due to the cancer.

We held hands and prayed. Specialists kept a watchful eye on Victoria, and right on schedule in September 2006, our miracle boy, Sidney, was born — big, beautiful, and healthy.

Soon after, Victoria had her left breast reconstructed and her hair grew back nice and curly. When she ran her hands through it and made silly faces, I began to see my old Victoria returning.

Life was good until the winter of 2007, four months after Sidney's birth, when Victoria stood in the bathroom one morning, wrapped in a towel and frozen in shock.

"Honey, there's a lump under my right arm," Victoria said to me. "It can't be back, can it?"

I pulled her close. Her heart pounded against mine. I had to be strong for her sake and for the children. But inside, I was gripped with fear. How could a woman so young be stricken again? I put my head down and wept.

The ultrasound showed three lumps and later, twelve tumors. Victoria was diagnosed with Stage IV breast cancer. The chemo affected her much worse after the second mastectomy and her curly hair fell out with the very first treatment. And she was perpetually tired.

"I can't get down on the floor and play with Amira. I can't bounce Sidney on my knee. I'm not much of a mommy, am I?" She was lying in bed, a scarf wrapped around her head, her gaunt face showing the effects of her battle.

"Shhhh, you're a great mom," I said. "Everyone is praying for you. Save your strength for the fight." Fight she did, but the doctors rushed her to the hospital with a very low blood count. I walked in one afternoon and found her sobbing so hard it scared me.

"What's wrong?" I rushed to her side and began to cry myself.

"A pastor came into my room. We had a long discussion about God and hope. Do you think I can live a long life? Do you think that's possible?"

"I absolutely believe you will live a very long life," I said. "We're going to grow old together."

Victoria put her head back against the pillow. "It's time to begin living without fear," she whispered. And then louder, and with conviction, "I'm going to look at every day as a good day to be alive."

She was soon released from the hospital, and gradually regained her strength. A few months later, I just had to ask her again.

"Victoria, will you please marry me?" I was down on bended knee, hoping for the answer I'd been praying for.

She fingered the scarf on her head. "I don't want to get married without my hair."

"You're beautiful. Marry me."

We locked eyes, hers searching and mine pleading.

"You know what?" she said. "Let's get married!"

On May 15, 2007, we celebrated Victoria's last chemo treatment.

"I made it," she said. "Again."

In July, we were bound together in a beautiful ceremony near the beach in Maui. The ebb and flow of the ocean reminded us of God's awesome power to heal, to restore our faith, and to rekindle hope. I lingered over a long kiss with my beautiful wife.

Every day is a good day to be alive.

~Charles Marshall as told to B.J. Taylor

27

Sorrow to Joy

noticed a woman across the room, looking pale and overwhelmed. It was our first breast cancer support group meeting. She'd just had surgery and was about to begin chemotherapy and radiation. I was in the middle of radiation treatments and beginning to feel the fatigue myself, and listening to stories of treatments, recurrences, and metastases was hard. And yet, there was a resiliency and strength in that room I couldn't quite understand.

It wasn't long before I grew so fatigued that I needed to leave before the meeting ended. The woman, who seemed to be growing paler and more drawn with every story, got up to leave at the same time and we walked out together. I said something about the difficulty of hearing all the stories. She responded, but we were both tired. I didn't see her again for six months.

I was depressed for days following that meeting. My colleagues, friends, and family all suggested I shouldn't go anymore if they affected me like that. But although it was unsettling, I was determined to sort out the discrepancy between the difficult stories and the positive aura of the group.

My colleague had a framed print in her office of a quote from Kahlil Gibran which helped me reconsider my situation.

"The deeper that sorrow carves into your being, the more joy you can contain."

Another friend of mine, and a breast cancer survivor, told me that making myself the priority would be vitally important for my treatment and recovery. As a mother and a clinical social worker, I'm very familiar with being "other" directed, but I didn't think I was doing such a bad job of taking care of myself, so I wasn't exactly sure what she meant. At the same time, I knew I wasn't okay. I knew my world had been turned upside down, and I knew I couldn't be there for others if I wasn't well myself.

I decided to work on giving myself permission to pay less attention to the world around me with all of its external stresses and demands, and work on allowing myself time to do what I needed to heal myself.

I began radiation treatment during a hot and humid summer. The staff drew what I considered to be a bad imitation of a Picasso (his blue period) on my chest to indicate the area to be radiated, and instructed me not to wash these marks off for the next seven weeks. Sounded simple enough, but they failed to mention that the blue latex paint would adhere itself to whatever clothing I wore and was anything but water resistant.

I began to look forward to tattoo day, when the radiated area gets marked permanently, assuming of course that after this was done I would no longer have to wear my Picasso. I was wrong. I took at least two showers a day with my back to the water, not only to protect the markings but to keep the direct force of the water from running on the radiated area. It was a challenge washing my armpits as I was not allowed to wear any deodorant on my radiated side.

After a few weeks of using cornstarch, I bought some deodorant whose only ingredients were seawater and minerals. I begged my oncologist to let me use it, and she approved. I was ecstatic. As personal grooming was beginning to take up quite a bit of my spare time I decided to use the structure of the daily radiation treatment as the impetus for taking care of myself.

First item on the agenda: buy an electric razor and shave my armpits. Next, I bought several frivolous beach books and a bunch of CDs. I couldn't remember the last time I had bought a CD or recreational book for myself. I listened to music in the car every day as I drove myself to treatments and I brought a book to read in case I had to wait. Both became calming and soothing rituals.

I worked on allowing myself to do what I needed to do.

I cried in the sanctity of my bedroom. I went to see Bill Cosby and laughed until I thought I would bust something. I went to football games. I bought myself a real Coke, not the diet kind, as my treat. I made very few plans and stayed close to home on the weekends and rested and relaxed. I allowed myself not to feel bad because I was too tired to go out.

And I refused to be robbed of my sexuality. I made love to my husband passionately and it helped me feel alive and escape how scary my life was. And when I would start to cry or get upset when it was not appropriate, I had a funny memory that would make me smile. I would remember the irony of the anesthesiologist telling me, as I was lying on the hospital gurney about to be wheeled in for breast cancer surgery, that I was an "extremely healthy woman" and as I just laid there looking up at him thinking, "What, are you nuts?" he added, "Well, except for the breast cancer."

I gained a new appreciation for life. I became aware that I wasn't going to live forever and that I needed to be choosier about how I spent my time. I made a commitment to continue to relax and to live it in a way that has more meaning. My cancer diagnosis has given me the opportunity to examine and reevaluate myself and I am better for it.

When the woman I watched at that first meeting returned six months later, I barely recognized her. She was exuberant and animated as she told her story and display her newly growing hair. She looked and sounded great. As a teacher, she was able to use her experience positively in her classroom, teaching awareness, respect, and compassion for others. What a turnaround it had been for both of us.

Khalil Gibran was right. All that sorrow had produced great joy.

~Christine Durbin

28

Chicken Soup for the Soul

Harder on the Patient or the Spouse?

When my wife was diagnosed with breast cancer, it was hard on her. And it was hard on me. So who had it worse? That may seem an absurd question, yet I've heard more than a few breast cancer survivors proclaim, "It's harder on my husband than it is on me." Let me give you my perspective.

In 2001, my wife was diagnosed with bilateral breast cancer—a lump in each breast. I tried to be the best caregiver I could be. Being a typical guy, I screwed up. I played the denial game. I tried to cheer her up relentlessly. Eventually, I got the hang of how to help (in a nutshell: don't try to fix things, just shut up and listen).

I certainly endured a lot of emotional pain. I remember the nights right after the diagnosis when I'd fall into a heavy sleep and never want to wake up, because waking up meant it was time to jump back into our war on cancer. We were busy fighting our HMO for referrals to "out of network" breast cancer specialists. We ran from one doctor's office to another. As days turned into weeks, I often found myself sitting in a waiting room while my wife was undergoing assorted surgeries. I'd watch *The Price Is Right* on the TV mounted high on the wall and wait and wonder what was going to go wrong (or right). And wish it were all as easy as guessing the cost of a new tube of toothpaste.

I felt as if I were balancing a plate on one upstretched arm. Upon that plate was piled: Marsha's breast cancer diagnosis; a report of suspicious cells that appeared to be a lymphoma, which caused the surgeon to say, "Boy, you guys just can't catch a break"; a big heaping of fear of the unknown; and a practical side dish of worry about whether we could make it financially if Marsha had to take a medical leave from her teaching job. On top of that, there were the usual pressures from my job and the daunting task of raising two teenage daughters.

I was petrified that I was going to drop the plate. I thought I was going to melt down in a weeping heap, unable to function. Who could I confide in? If I exposed my panic to Marsha, surely I'd be burdening her at a time when she had enough to deal with.

But I didn't drop the plate. As time went by, I learned that my arm—and spirit—were stronger than I'd thought. I also realized that selfishness is key in coping. A cancer caregiver isn't on call twenty-four hours a day. I made time for things I like to do and those precious moments helped me cope. With my wife's permission, I went for long jogs and longer bike rides; I lay on the floor in yoga classes and followed a yogi's commands; I spent hours in front of the TV watching silly DVDs. Even work could be a balm. When Marsha was going through chemo, weekends were hellish: She was upstairs in bed, feeling crappy; I was juggling the jobs of caregiver, errand-runner, and dad. When I'd get to work on Monday, I'd settle into my office with a sigh of relief. For the next eight hours, I'd know what I was doing and I even got an hour off for lunch.

In short, I could escape. And that eased the crush of cancer.

But what about the toll on Marsha? While I was watching TV in the waiting room, she had two surgical biopsies, then had a cancerous tumor sliced out of each breast. A drain stuck in her armpit caused excruciating pain. She endured countless pokes and pricks. Six chemotherapy sessions caused her hair to fall out and made her feel as if she'd just stepped off the world's craziest roller coaster (and she is a woman who cannot even tolerate a merry-go-round). A port was implanted in her chest to ease the delivery of chemo drugs but it caused a blood clot that made it hard for her to breathe and made her face all puffy from fluid retention. She could barely walk down the hall at the school where she teaches without getting winded.

Yet during her five months of chemo, she dragged herself to work just about every day, even though she was often wobbly and weary. Work distracted her, she later told me. At home, she'd just worry about the cancer: Did the surgeon get it all? Would chemo and radiation work their magic?

And, what if they didn't?

Marsha had to face her own mortality, which is a heck of a lot more daunting than what I had to face: the unspoken "what if" that hovers when a loved one has cancer.

Unlike me, Marsha never really could escape all of these worries, because her body always reminded her of what she was going through.

I could sympathize with her traumas. But I couldn't even begin to imagine the courage it takes to submit to the seemingly endless (and endlessly painful) treatments. I'm not sure I would have been as brave as Marsha. During her chemo months, I had a dream in which I had to have a chemotherapy infusion. I was a total chicken. I wouldn't let them stick that needle in my veins. I awoke in a cold sweat. But it was just a dream.

So, was it harder on me than Marsha? I think not.

She makes no bones about it: She believes her cancer was hard on me but harder on her, then and now. Even seven years after her diagnosis, she carries all sorts of scars, dents in each breast, fingernails that break more easily, and the notorious chemo brain. She's sure she's got it: a diminished ability to juggle many tasks and details.

I once trudged on a thirty-mile cancer walkathon, partly to get an inkling of Marsha's cancer ordeal. Afterward, nursing my blisters, I asked her if I could ever really understand what she went through. She smiled the wary smile of those who have endured a lot and simply said, "There's just no way."

~Marc Silver

29

Chicken Soup for the Soul

Cancer
Through My Eyes

February 1, 2005, is a day I will always remember. I woke up with a feeling that, one way or the other, my life was going to completely change, and I was right.

For the past four days, I had been trying to live my normal day-to-day life. I was an energetic eighteen year-old girl who had just started her spring semester at the college of her choice, Kent State University. As an interior design major with great friends and a fun job, I was extremely content and pleased with my developing life. Like every other young person, I was trying to discover my role in this world and had a feeling that things were coming together.

I called my mom, Lisa, after class and nervously asked, "Have you heard anything yet?"

"No, nothing," she replied.

We were awaiting the results of a biopsy, which had been done because of a tumor in my chest that was discovered when I went to the emergency room to have an egg-sized, mysterious lump on my neck checked out.

That night in the emergency room was filled with uncertainty and fear. I had never been to the hospital, so it was truly scary. The friends I called were as shocked as I was.

More testing led to more doctors but no results. After many

exhausting and confusing consultations, I finally found a doctor who wanted to do the biopsy. A few days later, I was waiting all day for his call.

February 1, 2005, was the longest day of my life. It was like being a kid and waiting several hours in line to get on a ride at an amusement park. In both those situations, you could feel nervous, excited, impatient, and scared. I was all of those emotions wrapped into one.

I went home after school and my mom called to let me know that she would be home shortly from work and that she would be bringing a family friend with her. I thought nothing of this at the time but it makes perfect sense to me now. She brought Stan, a great family friend of ours. She sat me down on the couch and said, "I heard from the doctor. The biopsy concluded that you have cancer."

Cancer? What could she possibly be talking about? My mom proceeded to tell me that I had Hodgkin's Lymphoma and that the doctor said that if I were to get any type of cancer, that was a good one to get.

"A good one?" I asked. "Why?"

She said that it had a very good cure rate and that I was going to be fine.

Going to be fine? A good cure rate? Were we really talking about this?

Just a few days before, I was a perfectly healthy young woman and now there I was, talking about if I was going to live or not. All of these questions started to pop into my head and then I went completely blank. I don't remember a lot from the rest of that evening except calling my brother, Adam, and a few friends to give them the news. The silence on the other end of each phone call was too much to bear. We all went to sleep that night with questions, confusion, and shock.

Within a few days, I met my oncologist and had several more tests. My doc diagnosed me with Hodgkin's Lymphoma, Stage IIb. He told me that I was going to have twelve chemotherapy treatments, each two weeks apart. I had to withdraw from school because I could not do both. The day I withdrew from school was difficult because instead of feeling like a young, vibrant woman, I felt like a sick, cancer patient who had to give up important things in her life.

It was all happening so fast. My mom accompanied me to each and every chemotherapy session. I had the best team of nurses and doctors behind me. They were always willing to do anything to keep us as comfortable as possible and were always open and honest.

As my treatment went on, everything changed, from my appearance to my relationships. I didn't feel like a young woman anymore and was out of touch with many people in my life. My doctor referred me to a local cancer center called The Gathering Place. Through this amazing organization, I was able to find a group of young people just like myself. I started going to the support group as often as I could and realized that I was not alone in this journey. Just when I thought I was alone, I learned that I was not.

After struggling through twelve treatments and countless scans and blood withdrawals, I finally finished treatment. Pending the results of my last CT and PET scan, I would have the opportunity to go back to school.

In August 2005, we found out that there was still active cancer in my body and additional treatment was needed. It was another crushing day for me because I wanted to get back to my old life. Within a few weeks, I started low-dose radiation treatment that lasted for about a month.

Finally, just before Thanksgiving, I received the news from my doctor that everything looked clear on my scan. On that day, I felt like I could finally get back to my old life, but there was something that felt weird about it. Even though I was clear of cancer, I realized that I could not go back to the life I once had. My friends had changed; my family had changed; my job had changed, and even where I lived had changed. I hadn't realized it as much while I was in treatment because the focus was elsewhere, but when it was finally over, I realized that everything was different.

I went back to college at a new school, Cleveland State University, where I am currently working on my undergraduate degree in psychology and have great hopes for the future.

I have learned several important life lessons from my cancer experience and feel lucky to have learned them at such a young age. I am currently a twenty-two-year-old woman and often feel old beyond my years. I have learned to keep the people that I love very close and informed, and if there are people in my life who cannot be with me through the worst, then they really did not deserve to be here in the first place.

Through my friends at The Gathering Place, I have learned how to live, love, and enjoy each day, because each one is truly a gift. Losing several dear friends from there has taught me what life is really about. I have learned not to take life so seriously, even though that can be easier said than done. I have learned that it is important to take time for yourself and to spend as much time as possible with the ones you love.

Even though my treatment is complete, my journey with cancer is not. I am still learning how to balance being a young woman who is finding her way in the world and is also a cancer survivor. This balance is something that I will always be searching for, as cancer did change my life for the better. I am hopeful that I will find my balance one day.

~Amy Chmielewski

30

Cancer Cell Beater

We have all lived through it—watching close friends or relatives slowly decline as a malignancy robs them of their vitality and quality of life. All of the treatments available have been tried, some may have helped for a while, but now the tumor has become resistant to every modality the doctors attempt. All we are left to do is watch this shadow of the person we used to know as healthy grow weaker by the minute. It makes us feel helpless, hopeless, angry and heartbroken, for soon they will no longer be with us.

It's a long way from a loved one's bedside to the small biopharmaceutical company in Malvern, Pennsylvania, where my colleagues and I are working to discover and develop a new class of drugs to treat cancer. We, like many dedicated scientists in other large and small pharmaceutical companies, devote our lives to the hope that one day our new medicines will help alleviate the suffering cancer brings. The idea that our drugs may make it possible for a young mom to be reunited with her children, a father to come home to play baseball with his kids, or a young child to grow up to be a happy and healthy adult is why we come to work each day.

Every day, fifty to seventy billion cells are instructed to die in our bodies. This is a necessary process that allows healthy new cells to replace aging ones. The process of cells dying is a highly controlled one that is called *apoptosis*, which is a Greek word that means "petals dropping off a plant." Apoptosis is defined as "programmed cell death" since it must be a highly regulated process. If too many cells die, it can result in a disease like Parkinson's or A.L.S., and if mutated cells that should die do not die as directed, the result can be cancer.

One of the ways that tumor cells cheat death is by making more proteins called IAPs (Inhibitors of Apoptotic Proteins). These proteins effectively block the signals the tumor cells are given to die. With the cell death pathway effectively blocked, the tumor cells are able to keep growing and mutating into an ever more deadly tumor. One strategy to remove the cell death block is to attack the IAPs in the tumor cells. Our company of twenty scientists set out to make a drug that did just that.

It was not too many years ago that cancer chemotherapy consisted of severely toxic drugs that indiscriminately killed healthy normal cells as well as tumor cells. These drugs killed normal, healthy rapidly dividing cells in the intestinal track and elsewhere in the body at the same time as the tumor. The end result was horrendous side effects and for many patients, death.

The last decade has witnessed the emergence of a new class of anti-cancer drugs called targeted therapy. These drugs target specific vulnerabilities in specific tumors. The days of one treatment for all cancers are numbered as more of these new classes of drugs emerge. The bright future of cancer chemotherapy is one where the unique properties of every patient's tumor will be characterized before treatment starts and a specific combination of drugs that target each tumor's vulnerabilities will be chosen.

My twenty-eight years in the pharmaceutical industry have been in companies both big and small, including the last two that I helped to start. The path from a good idea to an approved drug is a very long and torturous one filled with unexpected positive and negative surprises along the way. When working in an area of unexplored biology, you can never be too sure of what result is around the next corner. You form hypotheses and test them. Sometimes, the outcome is what you expect and some of the time it is a complete surprise. You make thousands of novel new compounds in the laboratory, evaluate them over years in a range of tests, and take the best one forward to test with patients.

Over the ten to twenty years it takes to bring a new class of medicine from an idea to a drug in the pharmacy, you oscillate between the elation of a seeing a radical response in a patient who failed all previous therapies to the devastation of obtaining a negative result which makes you question if you can ever get the drug FDA approved. After years of work, a promising new medicine can be stopped in its tracks by one significant negative result. As a result, it's back to the drawing board to find a new compound with improved properties that can meet the high standards that the companies and the FDA set in order for a drug to be sold commercially.

These days, the average cost is nearly one billion dollars to get a drug through years of rigorous testing. Throughout the dramatic roller coaster ride that drug discovery and development takes us on, there is one thing that keeps me and my colleagues going: the thought that the work we do might change the outcome for all the cancer patients who have just been told there is nothing else that can be done.

~Mark McKinlay, PhD

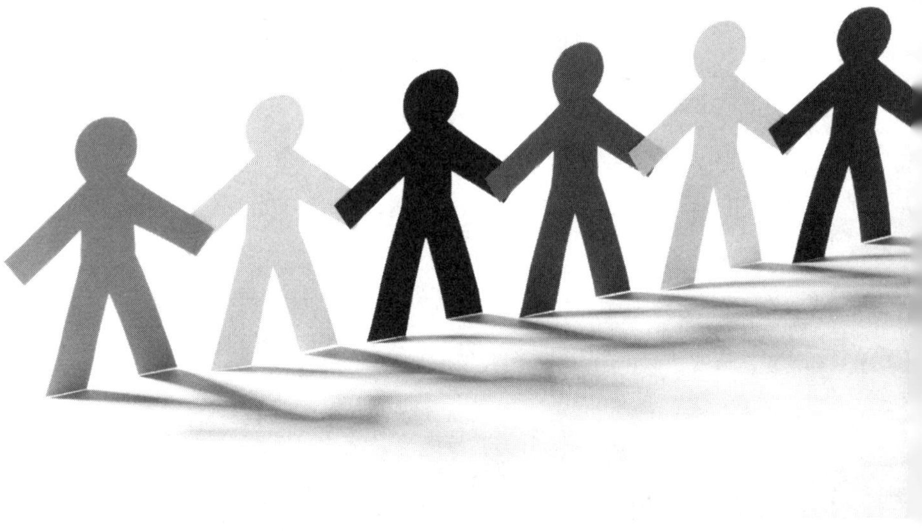

The Cancer Book

Unfinished Business

Perseverance brings good fortune.

~I Ching

31

Chicken Soup
for the
Soul

My Cancer Triathlon

I awoke from my first colonoscopy exam to hear the five words no one wants to hear.

"You have a cancerous tumor."

I was initially more distressed about the possibility of needing a colostomy than dealing with Stage III colorectal cancer.

My surgeon's goal was to alleviate the blockage in my colon before surgery and to ease the side effects of radiation and chemotherapy. She promised me "better living with a colostomy."

After my initial diagnosis, I'd been enjoying the blissful delusion that a quick surgery would take care of everything. I'd recover during Christmas break and return to teaching just after New Year's Day. Who would have thought that it would prove to be just a warm-up compared to what was coming?

I'd been propelled into the cancer triathlon: radiate, medicate, and operate.

I wasn't prepared for this endurance contest. I am grateful that my family, friends, and co-workers jumped in to help me get in shape for the race of my life.

But first, I needed a cover for my colostomy bag that would feel soft and not so sweaty. Since my version of sewing includes a stapler and duct tape, I was particularly grateful that my husband, Mark, had the skills to sew me a customized colostomy cover. He turned a well-worn flannel pillowcase into a soft bag, complete with Velcro fasteners. The diamond on my wedding ring may sparkle, but nothing compares to soft flannel next to my skin.

I was ready for the first milestone—a tattoo on my backside. The radiation staff wanted a marker to focus their beam. I hoped I wasn't setting a precedent and told my children this was no reason for them to get one, too.

For six weeks I attended a new spa treatment center I called the "Cancer Clinique." Two attendants enthusiastically greeted me each morning and had me lie face down on a white linen sheet before giving me my unique treatment. After I'd exposed my delicate areas, they demurely draped me with a towel and the whirring began. A slight sense of warmth enveloped me and then it was time to go. I was getting a sunburn but without the benefits of a total tan. I've always enjoyed the sun, but I'm no longer appreciating the effects of radiation.

Simultaneously, I began training for my second event—wearing a chemo pump for forty-two days and nights. Although it fit in a fanny pack and the infusion lines hid discreetly under my clothes, attached to the port in my chest, living with a pump 24/7 wasn't easy. Try sleeping with a three-and-a-half pound metal pack around your waist or showering while tethered to a three-foot line.

And the chemo drug itself was no picnic. It's abbreviated as 5-FU. (What can I say? The name says it all.) Perhaps the drug marketers should disclose what it really means: fatigued, flue-like, frail, frazzled, and fearful.

Like all athletes, I needed a break from training. My friend gave me a ticket to the U.S. Men's Ice Skating Championship in Spokane, WA. I was enjoying a night of superb skating when during the first intermission I heard a strange, beeping sound. My chemo pump was in alarm mode and the screen message kept blinking.

"High tension." Was that describing my blood pressure or the machine?

I called my home health care nurse.

"Get home immediately; there might be a clot."

Normally, the chemo pump has a reassuring click and whirring sound that goes off every hour. But at that point it sounded like a muffled ambulance siren going off every minute during the eighteen-mile drive back home. Thankfully, it was just a kink in the electrical line.

Earlier in the week, I'd purchased a "Chocolate Crisis Center Meltdown Bar."

Who knew it would come in so handy? I soothed myself munching on chocolate while watching the rest of the skating routines from my couch.

After completing the radiation and chemo components, I prepared for my third event—the big surgery. I e-mailed everyone I knew to ask for prayers, especially the SOS prayer, also known as "Save Our Sphincter." Not only was my surgeon going to remove the cancerous tumor and do a hysterectomy, she was optimistic about re-attaching my colon. After living with a colostomy for six months, I was hopeful too.

My biggest job had been to run the race the best way I could. Now, it was time to let God handle the rest.

I'm grateful for a successful surgery and for a surgeon with small hands to maneuver in tight places. Most of all, I appreciate my support team. Triathletes get all the attention, but it's those behind the scenes who make their participation possible.

~Susie Leonard Weller

32

Chicken Soup
for the Soul

Still Climbing

've been through a lot in my life and I'm still trying to figure out what it means.

When I was thirteen, I was diagnosed with advanced Stage IV Hodgkin's Disease and told I was going to die within three months. My body swelled from the medicine and I was unrecognizable to my friends and family. However, regardless of how I looked, I managed to survive and go on with my life.

About a year later, while in remission, I was diagnosed with yet another, completely unrelated cancer and given fewer than fourteen days to live.

Unimaginable.

At that point, my future only consisted of each day that I woke up. Tomorrow was barely available as an option.

Consider how much you've accomplished in the past two weeks, or for that matter, what you haven't done simply because you've been tired or too lazy or too scared.

Time is relative.

I was placed in a medically induced coma for nearly a year, undergoing intense treatment and radiation, leaving me with one functioning lung.

I've seen the world from the lowest point and from its highest — literally — as the first cancer survivor to climb Mount Everest. Although I took everyone touched by cancer to the top with me—scribbled on a flag and etched in my heart—I didn't have to reach the top of the world to find what I was looking for. I had only to look into my heart and listen to my soul and realize what they were already telling me.

Sean's true yearning for love? Hmmm, sounds like a weepy afternoon movie.

But don't be fooled into thinking I'm just a big pansy, because I'm probably more rugged than most people. (If you don't mind, I'll boast about climbing 29,035 feet with one lung, climbing the highest mountain on each continent, surviving altitude-induced swelling of the brain and being given my last rites by a man of the cloth as well as finishing the Hawaii Ironman.)

I appreciate what I've been given and I don't want to lose out on anything life has to offer. My experiences have taught me that one way to go through life is to make mistakes, fall flat on my face, and fail, only to get back up, dust myself off and continue forward with the knowledge of why I failed. Next time around it won't happen again because I believe that old cliché is right: "Those who fail are those who refuse to try."

After I went into remission for the second time, I wasn't afraid of anything.

I wasn't even afraid of girls, unlike practically every boy I knew. Nope. Why should I?

Would they kill me, like cancer had tried to do—twice? Did it matter to me if some strange girl didn't want to go out with me? Ha. Hell no. I'd been through so much more.

One person's opinion, no matter how cute she was, didn't bother me one bit. I took so many chances with girls when I was in college because what did it truly matter? My life was no longer in jeopardy and after worrying about whether or not I'd actually live through the night and wake up alive the next morning, I didn't care about some random girl saying, "No."

But I also learned that once I actually was in a relationship, it took a while to warm up and be honest with her about my cancers. Why? I have no idea. I thought maybe she'd see me differently or she'd be scared of me for some reason. Maybe she'd feel sorry for me, or maybe she just didn't want to be with someone who had been so sick, as if I might start all over again at any minute.

When I had started college, no one knew who I was. It was my opportunity to start over and not be known as "cancer boy." I didn't tell any girls I'd had cancer until I had dated them for a while. Finally I'd ask them if they were comfortable with me and who I was and whether they would hold it against me if I had a secret in my past. Actually, being a cancer survivor was probably much better than what might've been going through their minds regarding my secret life, so when I finally did tell them, they let out a sigh of relief!

I gave my heart freely back then and, in spite of everything I've lived through, I still do.

~Sean Swarner

33

In Her Honor

Six years ago, at the tender age of twenty-seven, my sister, Amy, was diagnosed with bone cancer. At first, she was reluctant to create a CaringBridge website to keep family and friends informed, because she didn't think anyone would want to hear about her day-to-day struggles. But within minutes of creating it, she was calling me to report that twelve people had already left her a guestbook message!

Watching the traffic to her website continue to grow became an addiction. What was even more amazing was the support our family gleaned from all the guestbook entries. Friends and family members from all over the world stopped in, thought about us, and then left a heartfelt message.

Amy was all about facts in her journal entries, listing details of her chemo regimen, blood counts and transfusions. She wanted everyone to understand her disease and its treatment. Her dry and twisted sense of humor, even about lab work, a tumor removal, and knee replacement surgery, kept everyone laughing and engaged.

Those of us who checked in on Amy each day became a tight-knit group. We were all pulling for my sister. On the good days, we cheered her on, celebrating small victories. On the bad days, we lifted her up, encouraging her to believe that she would get past this horrible time in her life.

Amy and I had pretty much been inseparable since the day

she was born. I was nine years older, and to me, she was "mine." I changed her diapers, fed her, and played with her, nonstop. My parents thought she had been sleeping through the night since she was two weeks old, when in fact I was getting up with her to give her a bottle every night. Eventually, they had to sit me down and break it to me that she wasn't my daughter, and that it wasn't my job to be her sole caregiver. I let them believe I agreed, but I knew in my heart I would never, ever stop taking care of her.

We grew up as best friends. We never fought once in our lives. We adored each other. From day one, she made me feel like the most important person in the world. So, when she got sick, nothing changed. Even though she was twenty-seven, I wasn't about to stop taking care of her.

Amy lived four hours away and I couldn't always be with her, so I clung to her through her CaringBridge site. I checked in constantly from anywhere that had a computer. At night, when my family had gone to sleep and the house was quiet, I logged in to recap her day. It became my ritual. Each night, I celebrated or cried, based on the latest update. I thanked God for that vital connection.

There were times when Amy was just too tired or sick to enter the latest news so she would ask me to do it for her. I was honored to be her spokesperson. CaringBridge became the glue that held our family together. It was a place to not only report information but to share our hopes and the fears. It also became the place where family members we hadn't heard from in years were able to say, "we're here." The love and support were amazing.

Amy never talked about her prognosis. She believed wholeheartedly that she would beat cancer and move on with her life. But each chemo treatment made her sicker than the last, and her body was taking longer and longer to recover. More often than not, my mind would wander to that scary "what if" place and I would panic. There was just no way I could imagine my life without her.

Many around us refused to believe me when I'd tell them she was really not doing well. Many didn't consider her illness life-threatening and didn't want to hear any bad news. Human nature, I guess.

But the unthinkable, unexpected thing that no one wanted to talk about did happen. After nine months, Amy died.

I knew my life would never be the same.

When I numbly updated her CaringBridge site, I knew that those who loved Amy and dropped by regularly to leave a message would be stunned. She had never let on in her journaling that her prognosis wasn't very good or that her body just wasn't handling the chemo. Yet even in death, CaringBridge was there for us—relaying visitation and funeral arrangements and serving as a place to memorialize our precious girl.

Those who have lost a loved one understand fully what happens when the funeral is over and family and friends go home. Life resumes and everyone goes about their business. There's suddenly nothing to do. You no longer have to care for a sick loved one; there aren't calls to make or meals to cook, and you're left with ugly, raw emotions and a huge, cavernous hole in your heart.

Many mornings I would wake with a jolt, worried that I hadn't yet called Amy or checked her website to see what her blood counts were. It took weeks for me to realize there was no reason to do that and that she was gone. I could no longer take care of her.

There were nights I would spend hours reading her previous journals. I clung to a place on the Internet that Amy loved—a place where she shared her humor, her life, and her love. She loved CaringBridge and the support it had offered her and our family.

I decided that I needed to give something back—for both of us.

I wondered if there was any way I could volunteer. When I realized that CaringBridge was located in the same city where I lived I immediately sent an e-mail offering my time. Within minutes I received a response from the founder and executive director of the organization. Before I knew it, I was scheduled to help process donations at her house. I felt comforted, knowing that Amy would appreciate what I was doing.

I went back the next week and the one after that and the one after that. I initially volunteered because it was a way to feel close to Amy. That position turned into part-time contractor work, and in 2006, I proudly accepted a full-time job.

I have been on the receiving end of CaringBridge, and I understand the overwhelming support it brings. Now, I am on the giving end, and it is wonderful to be a part of the team that makes it possible.

I tell people that I work at CaringBridge because it feels good to do good.

Do I also work there to honor Amy? Absolutely!

~Kelly Espy

34

Chicken Soup
of the Soul

Eat Pie

My wife, Chris, received a renewal notice for a health and nutrition newsletter that she has been receiving for years. I asked Chris if she wanted to renew and she told me to give it to her. She brought it back to me a few minutes later with a note she had written:

I've always loved your newsletter and followed what it said.
I got breast cancer anyway.
So, now I don't read any health material and I eat pie.

Thanks anyway,
Chris Balch

I laughed out loud. "You want me to send this?"

She said, "Yes, send it just like that!"

I started to say something and stopped.

I remembered when Chris had her lumpectomy and the surgeon couldn't remove the whole tumor, which meant that she was going to have to have a mastectomy.

"The five-year survival rate for someone with your type of cancer and the stage you're in and the fact that it's spread to your lymph system is about fifty to sixty percent," her doctor told her.

Chris went pale. "You mean I only have a 50-50 chance of living for five years?"

On the way home that day, she cried. In a voice I'd never heard her use before, she said, "I don't want to die. Why is this happening to me?"

It absolutely broke my heart. I couldn't hold or comfort her because she was in the back seat. My eyes teared and I had to concentrate on driving, but I knew that I had to say something. Or did I? Everything that I considered saying seemed hollow, empty, or just plain stupid. What could I possibly say? I couldn't tell her it would be okay, because I didn't know that and she knew that I didn't.

I just listened to her cry. It was one of the hardest things I've ever done, but I'm convinced that, under the circumstances, it was the best thing.

• • •

And, when my instinct might've been to question her response to the health and nutrition newsletter, I held my tongue. Sometimes, the best thing you can do is nothing at all. So, that's what I did and we haven't heard from them since.

~Dave Balch

35

My Journey

've always wanted to travel. Each time I've journeyed to a new place, my thirst has increased. I want to explore unknown lands and visit friends around the world. I've never been to Asia, Africa, or South America. I want to know this world I live in and to discover other belief systems. I've made plans to do that, perhaps to even leave the planet.

But one should really be careful what one wishes for. Everything may happen differently than what one plans because while human beings think, God guides.

In July 2007, I began a new, thoroughly uncalculated journey when I sensed a pang and a pinch under my shoulder and in my left breast. The thought of cancer shot into my head. Panic. What should I do? Gynecologist! Mine had retired three years earlier and I was still searching for a new one. I tried in vain to secure an appointment but everyone was overbooked and didn't accept new patients, or only had dates available in three months, or they were on vacation—on their own trip.

Then, I remembered that my doctor of Chinese medicine and acupuncture was also a gynecologist. He immediately did an ultrasound. He thought it didn't look so bad, that it could be a fibroid but that I should have it tested further.

I was happy and relieved, as if a fat stone had fallen from my heart. I was relaxed, and I went on vacation. But before traveling,

I made an advance appointment with a doctor who had been well recommended. I left home feeling optimistic and ready to embrace a new experience.

When I returned, I went to my new gynecologist. She wasn't so optimistic and sent me to a radiologist. After a mammography and biopsy, I sat in her waiting room during my lunch hour, worried that she would tell me something bad.

"As you already thought, it doesn't look good," the radiologist said.

What could that mean?

"You have a malignant tumor in the left breast."

All the medical knowledge I had gathered from my physiotherapy education broke down at that moment. Is malignant good? How can a tumor be good?

Shock!!!!!

I heard myself talking to the doctor from someplace far away.

"I have cancer! What will I tell my mother?"

She lay in a hospital 700 kilometers away, awaiting a highly dangerous heart operation. Super great timing. How will I travel to two hospitals at the same time?

When I stopped crying and got myself under control, the doctor described my prognosis. Operation, chemotherapy, radiation: What steps should be taken? I was spinning on a carousel of too much information.

I took a long walk on the canal and got something to eat. I went shopping at my favorite boutique and bought very expensive clothing I couldn't really afford. What was I saving for, anyway? What's the point? If I felt miserable, the least I could do was look good. Everybody around me was laughing and enjoying life and I could be dead soon. I saw the movie of the end of my life, playing clearly before me.

There was something inside me that I could die from. I couldn't comprehend it. But one thing was clear: I had to act, and act fast.

I went back to work and, at some insane speed, took care of everything important. I suddenly managed double and triple my normal workload. I was clear and concentrated, much more so than usual.

I had to go into the hospital as soon as possible. Then what? Could I work again? When? I wanted to get back into everyday life. Would I be able to go back to work at all?

The time before the operation passed in a twinkling. At first, I didn't tell anyone anything. I needed to digest it for myself. The fear before the operation was big, at least as big as my uncertainty. I felt as if I were about to lose my purity—surely I had a few scars from life, but nothing like I was about to experience.

No matter what, one thing was clear. It was time to move into battle. The monster that was eating me up had to be taken out as fast as possible. Armed with cancer literature, relaxation and meditation techniques, visualization exercises, healing CDs, and natural medicines, I entered the hospital and began my newest journey.

The operation went well but none of the follow-up treatments sounded very tempting. I began mistletoe therapy and embarked on a long and difficult quest to make the right decision—allowing myself more time to decide or embarking on one of the many different treatment plans that everyone was suggesting.

"Listen to your heart," said my gynecologist, and I followed her lead.

No chemo, no radiation, and no anti-hormone treatment. I accepted only the antigen therapy, despite its many side effects.

I cleaned my house, in more ways than one. I began meditation and increased my yoga practice. Whether it helped to remove the cancer, I don't know, but it brought me calm and confidence.

I traveled to visit friends and family and took a magical cruise on the Nile.

At the same time, I investigated many possible forms of healing and listened to a medley of medical and spiritual alternatives.

• • •

Almost one year from my initial diagnosis, the cancer has returned, but my whole view has changed. I'm still here. And life is fun. I don't see cancer as an external monster. It's a part of me that I accept and I am not afraid of it anymore. It's even become clear that the cancer is helpful; it points things out to me.

I am still the same as before, but at the same time, I am surely no longer the same.

Cancer is an illness of our time. We are a people who throw carcinogens around our planet. We go selfishly on our way, no matter the consequences. So, whatever comes lies in the stars, in the hands of a higher power.

Once again, I am contemplating additional surgery, chemotherapy, and radiation, as well as anti-hormone and anti-gene therapies. My doctors and alternative practitioners have presented me with an intensive menu of choices. The final decision is mine. One single thing counts—that I go the way that makes me happy and believe wholeheartedly in my choice.

I don't know which way that will be but I am ready to continue the biggest journey of my life—traveling deep inside myself in search of healing, strength, and renewal.

After all, I have fantastic plans to go places I have never gone before.

~Daniela Palik

36

Red Mohawk

Getting a cancer diagnosis isn't easy to accept (I guess it never is), particularly when there isn't any real cure and you're given a life expectancy of one to five years.

Myelodysplasia.

Damn, I thought, I don't have time for that. I can't even pronounce it. I'm not ready to be sick, I don't even feel sick, and I'm a busy guy. I've got lots of stuff to do. I don't have time to waste with treatments and medicine and hospitals.

Like anyone who gets such ominous news, I immediately attempted to become an expert on the subject. I read all about the disease and I hoped I would stumble upon something my oncologist might have missed, something that would revolutionize my treatment and become a quick and easy fix.

Ha! I thought. I will hit the Internet, and in a matter of days I will know more than my doctor has learned in eight years of medical school.

The more I read, the more I found myself confused. But along the way, I learned enough to know what questions to ask my doctors.

I was initially sent to a treatment center for an experimental type of bone marrow transplant, but upon meeting the doctor, I felt uncomfortable with his approach. I went back to my original oncologist and had a frank discussion that basically boiled down to, "Which options give me a better chance of survival?"

He sent me to see another oncologist who specializes in conventional bone marrow transplants, a plain talking, no-nonsense guy with a logical approach. No experiments, no trials, just his success record for survival—sixty-four percent for guys my age with no other health issues. I didn't think those odds were too bad especially since I didn't have much of a choice.

We set the wheels in motion to find a bone marrow donor since none of my family members matched. I was feeling tired, weak, and out of breath but I had to keep working or I would lose my health insurance and my chance at a transplant.

You gotta love America!

After several months of frantic searching, a donor was located in Eastern Germany. I wondered how it could work, but it was worth a shot.

Preparing to travel out of state for a long stay in the hospital was a bittersweet moment. Friends and relatives dropped by to wish me well.

Were they coming to say goodbye?

Did they know something I didn't know?

Were they looking at me and saying to themselves, "dead man walking"?

I was freaked, but at the same time, I was determined to lighten the moment and relieve everyone else's stress. Maybe it would even relieve some of mine. I figured I was going to lose my hair at the hospital, due to chemotherapy and radiation treatments, so why not jump the gun? I decided to allow my twelve-year-old daughter, Alysia, to shave my head and save a big mess later when my hair would fall out anyway.

As a group of close friends and family watched, we sat in our front yard and Alysia and my wife, Lori, began to cut my hair. I was thinking about what a momentous event it was when Alysia blurted out, "Dad, let's make it a Mohawk!"

I weighed the pros and cons of walking into the hospital like that—a middle-aged man with a Mohawk about to risk his life in a bone marrow transplant—and I realized that this could be the final fun activity I would ever do with my daughter. I didn't want to disappoint her. It was her idea, and if that was how she was going to remember her dad, then that was how it had to be.

Someone ran to the store to get gel and red hair dye. Lori and Alysia clipped and shaved with renewed enthusiasm. My friends cheered as my fuzzy head became as slick as a bowling ball with a big chunk down the middle remaining uncut. Everybody got his or her hands full of gel, spiking my hair and adding red dye to color it. The final result wasn't as cool as what you see on people in the movies but we sure got our point across and had a blast doing it!

The next day, we headed to the Dana-Farber Cancer Institute in Boston to begin my quest for a new lease on life. It felt bizarre walking through Quincy Market as a tourist with a red Mohawk. I got a lot of stares at Fenway Park from Red Sox fans thinking, "Who is this middle-aged weirdo?" I guess I felt the need to show off my new hairdo and, with my family by my side sharing those stares, it was fun. We were having a blast even though I had a good chance of dying in the near future. (Although a sixty-four percent chance of surviving is a lot better than thirty-six.)

At the hospital, I became a novelty of sorts—the "guy with the red Mohawk." I don't know if I received any extra attention because of my hairdo, but people were always looking or stopping into my little, germ-free, bubble room.

My health care team quickly found me to be a proactive patient, well informed and determined to be an active participant in my treatments. The staff looked past my appearance and appreciated a patient who had a desire to learn and understand what was happening in his body. It made everyone feel better about my prognosis and eventual recovery.

This year, I will celebrate my sixth birthday, post transplant. I still count the days since the procedure. I am grateful for everyone who helped me get through this awful time, especially my little girl who first suggested I try a Mohawk.

~Spin Zucker

37

Chicken Soup for the Soul

Getting My Dad Back

"You have leukemia."

The doctor's words rang through my ears over and over again. I couldn't believe that my dad was diagnosed with cancer. At age ten, I wasn't even exactly sure what cancer really meant. I was speechless. My whole body felt numb. I couldn't cry or even speak. I just stood there like a ghost, with no connection to the world. I looked over at my mom, as a tear rolled down her cheek. How was I supposed to react?

My dad had just gotten a new job as a manager at CVS so luckily the insurance covered the bone marrow transplant. My dad's donor was a woman from Germany. After intense radiation and chemotherapy treatment to kill most of the cells in a patient's body, just before their immune system is about to die, the bone marrow is given intravenously and if the match works, the patient lives.

The day before my dad went into the hospital was beautiful. We spent the day outside shaving his hair into a Mohawk and dyeing it red. Most of my family came to visit him that day. He had a smile on his face as if nothing was wrong. I'm not sure if it was because he didn't want me to get scared and upset or because he never really let the cancer affect him. His attitude was admirable the entire time he was in the hospital and even when he came home. My mom and I visited him as frequently as we could.

Thinking about my mom and I kept him holding onto life, as

it was dangling on a thread for a long time. But my attitude wasn't as positive. Many days, I would get what seemed to be a large pit in my stomach. I was frightened by visions that I would walk into my house and find my mom crying and trying to explain to me that my dad died.

It was difficult visiting him because he was almost two hours away from our house. When I did get the chance, I dreaded being at the hospital. He literally lived in a bubble. His room was completely secluded from everybody else. He was never allowed to leave the room. When I wanted to see him I would have to thoroughly wash my hands and put gloves on. I couldn't enter the room without a hospital mask over my face. Not being able to hug, kiss, or even touch my dad was hard because he and I are so close.

Some days, he could barely answer my questions because he was so out of it from taking massive medication. As time went on, I watched my father grow weaker. He had barely any appetite so his weight dropped to 102 pounds and he is 5'8". Even if I could've given him a hug, he was all skin and bones.

Overall, my dad was in the hospital for four months. Before he came home, my mom and I had to get rid of our two ferrets because my dad had to be in a completely sterile environment while he was healing. We cleaned and bleached the entire house every day to make sure there were as few germs as possible. We got brand new furniture, which could be wiped down to eliminate mold and mildew. We also got new carpets to help eliminate dust particles.

When my dad first came home, he wore a mask and gloves until his body oriented itself to the environment. With all the medications and his catheters and masks it made my house feel more like a hospital than a home.

My mom worked night shifts, so I lived with close family friends. When I got sick during the school year, I had to move out because we couldn't take the chance of my dad getting sick. Many times, it didn't even feel like I had a home where I really belonged because I was always moving around so much.

It was weird getting used to my dad being around the house

so much because I was always used to him being away, working. I made him food when he was sick and I organized his medications. His catheters that were still surgically inserted into his chest needed to be cleaned every day, which I also usually did. Although it was sometimes difficult doing all of those things for my father, it helped us appreciate each other a lot more.

After about one-and-a-half years in the house, he was well enough to return to work. The doctors tried to limit his schedule to only thirty hours a week, but in order to keep receiving the insurance benefits he needed, he was required to work at least forty hours. The vicious cycle began again. My mom and I were used to it because he had always worked a lot. Soon enough, I barely ever saw him because I had school and he was gone most of the time.

Now six years cancer free, he works anywhere from sixty to seventy hours a week. He has gone from being so weak and so secluded from the world to working endless hours to support his family and to donating his time in the community.

My dad is amazing. As painful as it was to see him go through that period, it's even more rewarding to have seen him become the inspiring person he is today. I am so happy he is healthy now, able to enjoy his life and spend time with me again.

~Alysia Zucker

38

Chicken Soup for the Soul

Cinnamon Hearts and Rocky Mountains

Sunbeams pour in through the windows, warming the room and giving it a cheery atmosphere. In the distance, I can see the stately Rocky Mountains, appearing deceptively close in the morning mist. People lie in huge, comfortable reclining chairs, their voices soft and muted, interrupted by an occasional beep. Enjoying the taste of a tiny cinnamon candy, I sit and soak up the glorious vista before me.

Then, a quiet voice brings me back to where I really am, and why.

"Mom, can you please adjust the blinds? The sun is shining in my eyes."

Turning to my daughter, I notice the sunlight is directly in her face. As I rise to adjust the blinds, the reality of our situation pierces my whole being.

We're in a Treatment Room in a large Calgary hospital. Each of the large, blue chairs holds someone receiving intravenous therapy, enabling these people to regain their health and move on with their lives.

A young man studying the lines of a play in which he has a role is receiving a much-needed anti-rejection drug. A grandfather receiving blood transfusions has a photo of his grandson taped to the IV pole.

My daughter is receiving chemotherapy for the malignancy that has invaded her young body. Her purse holds an angel given to her by my sister to accompany her to treatments and various appointments.

The intravenous flow control pumps, so familiar to me from my years of nursing, hum, beep, and blink their miniature lights like futuristic, decorative trees. My daughter is settled in a chair at the end of the line, surrounded by her much loved books, yet constantly observing her fellow patients, chatting with her nurses, and occasionally reaching for her candy dish, filled with tiny red cinnamon hearts. A kind mother, whose son had undergone treatment, has told her that the cinnamon flavor will disguise the chemical taste caused by chemotherapy.

So many of those ailing people and their worried family members are sharing tips and stories. I've seen it often as a nurse and admired it so much. Now, the situation is reversed and I am the family member appreciating these tips, and my daughter is the patient.

We share anything helpful, anything that might ease the hurt for someone else. When I adjust the blinds, my eyes are drawn to the candy dish on the table connected to my daughter's chair. A tiny, dazzling sunbeam glistens off its shiny rim. The sun's warmth causes the red candy to emit the sweet smell of cinnamon. It's a smell of special occasions: mulled apple cider at Christmas time, stirred with a cinnamon stick, warm cinnamon rolls my daughter enjoys after skiing, and the smell of her favorite loaf I used to make. I decide to make it again soon.

As I remember these occasions, I am filled with heartache, but I won't let my daughter notice.

Never once have I heard her ask, "Why me?" I've never seen her be anything but pleasant to those she meets in this room or anywhere else in the hospital. She shares her cinnamon hearts, telling her fellow patients, "Mom got lucky, they're on sale after Valentine's Day," which makes those around her smile. I cannot help but admire her courage.

She is the young wife whose wedding pictures show a healthy, athletic, beautiful bride. She is the mother of a smart, equally beautiful three-year-old child, and she is my daughter who spreads words of encouragement to all she meets. I cannot help but be impressed at how patiently she sits for five hours while her life-saving medications are administered.

Peeking through the blinds a little later, I see that the mist has disappeared from the Rockies' peaks. The mountains look like the rock candy we had as children; the cinnamon hearts show their red blush and share their wonderful scent. Put it all together and it is a healing recipe for the soul.

I am in a room full of fear and courage, with a smiling, but very ill, daughter. And I have cinnamon hearts and Rocky Mountains. It is a moment to remember forever.

~Bonnie Jarvis-Lowe, R.N., Retired

39

Chicken Soup for the Soul

The Room of Hope

The Barcaloungers sit erect with their rigid arms permanently extended, as if in supplication, awaiting the next assortment of chemical bags to be draped upon them. The quiet in the large room seems incongruous to the fear and dread that will soon fill it. Each of the thirty small cubicles is equipped to make a patient comfortable while the fluids trickle slowly down the plastic tubes and into their veins. Muted sounds come from the TVs, distracting the patients as the hours pass slowly by.

The nurses move quickly from station to station, their soft rubber soles squishing on the linoleum. There is a calm to their work, but it still conveys an urgency and efficiency to get each of their patients properly tethered to their respective IV poles. They do this everyday with multiple shifts. It seems like an assembly line but they know that each patient is unique. They possess a gentle touch and soft words, with an expertise that says, "I will get you through this and make it as painless as possible."

Fear and depression accompany hope and optimism.

"Will I be sick?"

"Can I tolerate the drugs?"

"Will I lose my hair?"

"Is this the beginning of the end?"

"What will happen to my family when I'm gone?"

"Will I suffer?"

"Is there a realistic reason to be hopeful?"

"Can I get drugs to ease the side effects?"

"What do I do next if this fails?"

The list seems endless. Some questions have answers, but many do not. In spite of that, there is a tiny flame of hope that burns and refuses to be extinguished. It's resilient and pushes against the darkness. It takes nourishment from any and all victories, however small they may be.

"I made it through another chemo day."

"My scans are stable, no new growth."

"I have an appetite today."

"I was able to get up and take a shower."

"The birds are singing and the flowers look beautiful."

"My grandchildren are coming to visit."

Across this great country, in thousands of chemo rooms, patients struggle to survive. They seek the normalcy they were accustomed to before cancer. Sadly for most, their old lives are gone forever. The normalcy they seek is but a memory.

Is it better or worse than before? It is just different because the experience has made us that way.

Many of us have visited the chemo room. It was never a place to be enjoyed. The chemicals bring sickness and suffering. Many of us began the first step of our cancer journey right here. In most cases, it's lived up to its infamous reputation.

For me, with Stage IIIb melanoma, Stage I renal cell carcinoma and Stage I adenocarcinoma, it certainly has.

I believe that chemo rooms are truly rooms of hope, that the chemicals will do their job and kill the cancer cells, and upon completion of the chemo the scans will show that no evidence of disease remains. Chemo rooms offer the hope that the chemicals can slow down cancer's proliferation in our body and buy us some time. They offer hope that this drug will work after others have failed.

Hope does abound in a chemo room! Hope is the fuel and the

energy of our souls. Let us sustain and nurture the tiny flame of hope and keep the darkness at bay.

~Al Cato

40

My New Life

live in Canada, in a small town called Atikokan in northwestern Ontario, surrounded by lakes, rivers, and streams. We have a human population of about 3,000, and a mosquito population of three billion. At the present time, we have a huge black bear wandering the streets and making a nuisance of itself. It was spotted about six houses down from me last night. That's just one of the many benefits of living in the wild, like having the nearest fully equipped hospital three hours away by car.

I am a fifty-three-year-old woman. I have two part-time jobs and always thought I had all the time in the world to go on trips and take a holiday or to make things right and get in touch with old friends. I always thought I had all the time in the world to do the things you plan on doing — someday, tomorrow, next week, or perhaps next year.

In one day, with one phone call, my life has changed. I will never be the same person again and that is a strange, mixed-up feeling. I still have so much left to do!

I was too busy to visit the doctor on a yearly basis, too busy to listen to my body, too busy to be sick. Finally, I listened. My body was telling me that something was not right and I made an appointment for a physical. Ever since, I've been on a roller coaster of blood tests, urine tests, ultrasounds, and then, the phone call. They found a large tumor on my right kidney and are sending me for a scan to find out whether it is cancer or not.

I do not know what the diagnosis will be. To say that it does not matter would be a lie. Of course it matters, but probably not in the way most people would think.

When the doctor first called, I felt as though she had kicked me in the stomach. For a moment, I thought I would be sick. I definitely had to tell myself to breathe, and a million and one thoughts raced through my brain, fogging everything else she said after the word "tumor."

I realized I might not have all the time in the world, after all.

So, what do I do? I have decided I will live a fuller life, regardless of the outcome of my scan. Today, I will write a letter to my best friend and tell her how much her friendship means to me. Today, I will phone my sons and daughter, and tell them how very much they mean to me. And today, I will plant my flowers.

Is there a support group for people who wait?

• • •

The tumor is not in my kidney as they originally thought. I do not have kidney cancer. The tumor is confined to my adrenal gland, and as far as they can tell, there is no spreading. They will be removing the whole adrenal gland and doing a biopsy afterwards. It is my understanding that removing an adrenal gland is complicated, so I continue to have blood tests, urine tests, etc. Apparently, there is some medical preparation that needs to take place before this operation can happen; I am probably looking at two more months of waiting, depending upon whether this tumor is functioning or nonfunctioning. The doctor tells me adrenal cancer is very rare.

• • •

There is a certain amount of freedom in accepting what you cannot control. When I tried to explain this to my daughter, she became angry with me. I told her I was not afraid of death, just pain. I guess that is part of my faith. I have learned from this experience — no matter how much you and your family love each other, there are certain thoughts that are difficult to share, for whatever reason. Some of my family members do not mention the word "cancer." They do not ask me how I feel because I guess they are more afraid than I am of what I am going to say. My mother and I, on the other hand, have discussed all the possibilities, good and bad, and I appreciate her honesty.

• • •

Today, when I woke and my feet hit the floor, I thanked God for the good life I have had, and hopefully, will continue to have, and I realized I don't do that often enough. Today, I think about how I am going to live the rest of my life as a more loving, giving, and thankful person. Strangely enough, mixed in with all the other emotions I have at the moment, I have joy. All in all, I feel more alive than ever.

~Debra Manford

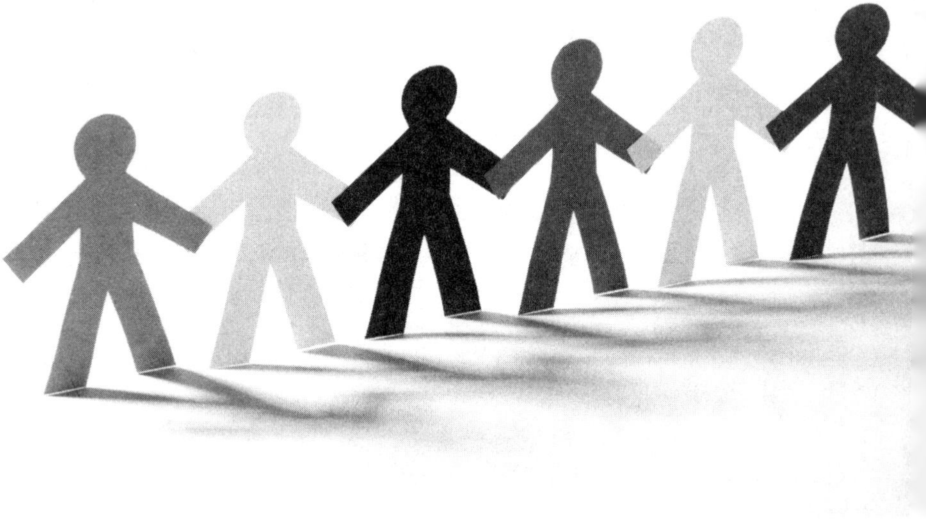

The Cancer Book

Dreams and Nightmares

Man is harder than rock and more fragile than an egg.

~Yugoslav Proverb

41

Chicken Soup
for the Soul

In the Ring

L ADIES AND GENTLEMEN! CHILDREN OF ALL AGES!
Welcome to the fight of a lifetime. Today, we host the
veteran heavyweight champion, Colon Cancer, taking on the
up-and-coming lightweight, a fierce competitor in her own right, Ali
Zidel Meyers.

Tonight's fight is brought to you by Zofran anti-nausea medication and the chemotherapeutic agents, Oxaliplatin, Leucovorin, and
Fluorouracil.

IN THIS CORNER, weighing in at an astonishing 7,000 pounds
and still growing: the indomitable, brain-numbing, throat-curdling
monstrosity of a fighter, Colon Cancer. C.C. has a deadly record,
standing with the likes of AIDS and heart disease as one of the high-
est-ranking foes on the planet. The much maligned, under-handed
killer has earned a wicked reputation among fighters of all shapes
and sizes across the globe.

This is cancer's 575-millionth fight.

IN THE OPPOSITE CORNER, weighing in at a petite 120
pounds, let's hear it for first-time contender, thirty-four-year-old Ali
Meyers, a feisty redhead from Columbus, Ohio, and mother of two
young children. She's a comparative lightweight, but she packs a
powerful punch. Her marathon-like endurance, agility, and stealth
intelligence have readied her for this monumental fight.

The anticipation is palpable, as both fighters step into the center of the ring, staring each other down.

AND THERE'S THE BELL!

Cancer throws a series of small jabs to the abdomen, while Meyers moves to block. Both fighters display colorful footwork, dancing across the ring. The air feels heavy, and Meyers wears a face of measured concern, as Cancer appears to be gearing up for one of its massive one-hit knockouts.

C.C. lands the first big punch! It's a massive blow to Meyers' abdomen. It appears that cancer has removed about a foot-long section of Meyers' ascending colon near the liver! The referee steps in to pull Cancer back as the cleanup crew clears oozing blood puddles from the ring. Meyers' intrepid surgical crew helps her up and sews her back together on the fly. The referee checks in with the Meyers team to see if the fight can resume. Meyers briefly panics as the realizations set in: she may die sooner than she planned; her once-hoped-for dreams may collapse before her very eyes.

BUT HOLD ON, LADIES AND GENTLEMEN! This is one tough cookie! Despite it all, Meyers climbs to her feet and with some creative patchwork around the belly, she resumes her stance with eyes ablaze. She's ready to rumble.

Meyers throws a punch to Cancer's trunk, followed by a surprise hit to the sternum. Cancer lunges forward. Meyers crouches low, averting a left hook, and as she shifts her feet, she appears to be gaining strength. Cancer seems momentarily confused. Meyers charges like a bull. She's in it to win it!

OH MY!! C.C. takes a sharp jab to the face. Meyers shocks Cancer with a fierce roundhouse to the head. Meyers is gathering momentum. The fight heats up. But Cancer recovers from Meyers' blows and seems to collect itself. C.C. motions Meyers to bring it on! The crowd leaps to its feet. The arena goes wild!

Meyers and Cancer are embroiled in a relentless, plundering scuffle. How long can this continue? The audience cheers and dances. As the rounds pile up, both fighters show signs of weariness; their once powerful punches diminish with each ring of the bell.

BUT WAIT A MINUTE, LADIES AND GENTLEMEN!

This is unprecedented. Colon Cancer is hugging Meyers and pulling on her shoulders, attempting to drag her to the ground. Cancer has started head-butting its opponent and appears to be lunging toward her kidneys. This is definitely against the rules. The crowd boos in disapproval. Meyers squats down and pulls back, escaping the embrace for the moment, as the referee steps in and calls a foul. Meyers' fans erupt as they witness Cancer's desperate attempts to overcome its target. The boos and hissing have drowned out the bell, signaling the end to yet another round of brutal fighting. Both Colon Cancer and Meyers retreat slowly to their corners.

Cancer looks for hydration and sustenance, but appears immobile and isolated. Cancer's team is absent. The trainer and medic have disappeared. Cancer looks disgusted, and its morale seems to be taking quite a hit.

In the opposing corner, Meyers loads up through her chest port with saline and a quick pump of high-dose Folfox. Oncology nurses swarm her as the doc checks her vitals and latest blood test results. Meyers stares across the ring at her opponent, pounding her gloves as the crowd chants, "Die Cancer die! Die Cancer die!"

As the clock ticks and the next round beckons, will cancer find the strength to step back in the ring? Will Meyers? Who will win? Nobody knows. Stay tuned, as the fight of a lifetime unfolds.

~Ali Zidel Meyers

42

Chicken Soup
for the Soul

Ode to Joy

One of the best parts about losing your hair from chemotherapy is the chance to get a new hairstyle or color. The wig store offers unlimited options. The place where I bought mine—aka my cranium prosthesis—had actual names for all of their products.

The wig I chose was labeled "Joy." This might seem like an oxymoron, considering my treatment for breast cancer, but I hoped it would be a prediction of things to come.

My daughter and I had great fun personifying the wig and referring to her by her name. If I walked out of the house, Joy accompanied me. She went to work, social gatherings, shopping, and church. I live in the windy panhandle of Texas, and some days it was a challenge to keep her from lifting off my head and blowing free, but she was always with me. When Joy and I came home, she went to her Styrofoam head, as I felt we both deserved a rest.

One day after work, and the appointment which concluded my second week of chemotherapy, I decided to clean my car. I went to Quick Quack, which cleans your car as you sit back and glide along. This seemed like a great idea, as my energy level was close to empty.

After the wash, I decided to vacuum the floor mats. Unfortunately, I parked a little too close to the mounted vacuum machine. I couldn't open my door but I was too tired to move the car. I figured I could squeeze into the tiny backseat and start vacuuming there. With a good deal of effort, I was able to manage that, and after wrestling with the hose to clean the front seat, I completed the job before my money ran out. However, by that time, I was exhausted and more than ready to go home. But I still had to get out of the car and return the vacuum.

The hose was still going strong, and because I was so tired, I struggled to get it out of my way and open the door. It was crowded in there, and hot, the hose was twisting over my mid-section and my patience was wearing thin. As I maneuvered myself into position to escape this predicament, I suddenly felt the desperate need to scratch my head. It was summer and Joy made me sweat. I only had one arm free to reach but I absent-mindedly lifted the vacuum up to my head. The hose instantly sucked Joy right off my bald, beautiful head. Obviously, I hadn't read the warning, explaining that the vacuum had a super duper velocity hose with enormous sucking capacity, urging all users to keep small pets and children away from it.

I wasn't surprised. I was shocked!

The darn thing wouldn't let go of Joy and my efforts to retrieve her seemed useless. She was halfway up inside the hose, stuck into the vacuum's throat, and I was struggling to reach up inside the thing and get her loose. For the first time ever, my quarters weren't running out and the vacuum kept running while both of us thrashed all over the back seat, fighting for possession of Joy.

Suddenly, I heard a very loud and hysterical laugh coming from the other side of the car. A man who had probably been watching the entire ordeal was standing next to his truck and laughing uncontrollably. When I first glanced over at him, he was holding his big belly with both hands, his face red from laughing and looking like it was going to explode. The more I struggled, the more he lost control of himself.

I am a person who normally loves to find humor in our daily lives, but in that moment I couldn't figure out exactly what was so darn funny about a bald woman wrestling with a super-sized vacuum hose, trying to retrieve the rest of her head.

As I finally excavated the last of Joy out of the vacuum, I saw that the man had tears falling from his face and he was trying to catch his breath. I very determinedly smiled and placed Joy hurriedly back upon my head, which started him all over again into convulsions of laughter.

Enough is enough, I thought. I frowned at him, and with as much dignity as possible, while trying to keep Joy in her place, I squeezed out of the small space in the back seat and got behind the driver's seat. As I glanced in the mirror, I caught a glimpse of Joy. I had inadvertently turned her upside down and that's when I lost it and started to laugh. I dumped the hose out of the back window, leaving it sprawled on the ground as I drove off, with a smile and a wave to my hysterical new friend. What a story he would have to tell his family when he got home.

As I repositioned my cranium prosthesis, I knew that my *Ode to Joy* would eventually bring smiles to others going through cancer.

~Charlotte Wheeler

43

Nuclear Medicine

This is the room where the body becomes transparent.
Walls of wires, computer monitors around a white table,
a man with a heavy apron and cold hands.
Everything bears the faint hum of electricity.

The leaded doctor lays me down, removes a syringe
from a lead-lined tube, and injects the isotope into my arm —
my veins feeling a sting of warmth.
I sleep the three hours it takes for my body to saturate.

My shoes on the table feel unwieldy.
The doctor swivels me over the white drum of a camera
and positions me onscreen for the dream of science, watching
the shape of myself coalesce to definition.

These are the black dots swirling in technology.
These are the cameras that see through
clothes, name, identity —
focusing on the dark, radiant pools of weakness.

In this room, I have had to let everything go.
The doctor directs me to look at the monitor,
points out the pelvic line, the bladder, black with radiation.

He lets the film scan everything I am —

rolling the table and its cargo up to view the spine,
the chest cavity ticking iridescently. I can do nothing
but be still, witness the monitor's ghost-images:
this heart, this black spot, this flickering.

~Nicholas Samaras

44

Chicken Soup
de the Soul

11:11

About twenty-five years ago, I began to notice that almost every time it was 11:11, I'd be looking at a clock. It was like I had a little secret without knowing why or what it meant, as if someone had told me a joke but I hadn't heard the punch line. For all I knew, I had a psychic connection with Timex.

When I was forty-three, married with two small boys, I was diagnosed with Stage II breast cancer. I was treated with a full mastectomy, chemotherapy, and immunotherapy.

My mother had died of colon cancer when I was a girl, so for me, cancer was utterly terrifying. Its scars were embedded in my psyche long before my own diagnosis. I'd worked for decades trying to heal from and resolve her death.

I thought of my mother all the time during chemo. When I lay on my bed, as I remembered her laying on hers, my son, then four, would come to play, but I was usually too wiped out to engage him. I thought of her when I couldn't carry my one-and-a-half-year-old boy while recovering from surgery. I remembered her when I'd ponder dying, as one must when faced with a potentially terminal illness. I came to accept the possibility of death in all areas of my life. Except my kids. Imagining myself dying and leaving my boys was a thought that burned so hot with fear I could only pray for mercy. How did my mother process her impending death that would leave nine children?

For the first time, I began to understand what she might've felt, leaving us when she died at age fifty. Beyond my painful memories, I developed a deep empathy for her, which opened up something in me that I didn't know was closed, as if the tears I was crying and the terror that trembled in me for my own life shook a pipeline clear.

I mostly lean away from believing in "other worldly" things. It brings to mind Dionne Warwick and the Psychic Friends Network. Growing up, whenever I'd hear people who had lost loved ones saying, "I miss her but I feel her every day. I know she's with me," I would thrash about in a sarcastic, jealous rage. I never felt my mother after she died. She was just gone. Gone.

Then, at the tail end of my treatment, I began to sense my mother's presence. I'd shake my head as though I'd fallen asleep by mistake, but it would happen again.

One day, while riding my bike, I was wearing a gold bracelet my mother had willed to me in a sort of dare that it could summon her. Sailing down a hill, I heard her "say", "I was lame." Luckily, I was alone, so I continued to "talk" to my dead mother.

"You were lame," I said back, painfully aware that she hadn't said goodbye or left me prepared in any way for her death.

Around this time, I reached out to my mother's only living sibling. Margie had begun calling during my cancer treatment for the first time ever, leaving messages of support and love. I was delighted and had to wink at the cancer for bringing her into my life. I felt an increasing need to visit her. She was eighty-six. It had to be soon.

Driving up to Boston on a sunny Sunday morning, I glanced down at the clock and it was 11:11. I smiled, as I always have at this quirky phenomenon. About forty-five minutes later, a mental coin dropped and I nearly swerved off the road. My mother died when I was eleven! Could that be what the 11:11 has been all this time? Has she been tapping at me all these years and I didn't get it?

I pulled into Aunt Margie's gravel driveway, my mind pulsating with elevens, and readied myself to see a woman who looks and speaks like my own mother, now dead thirty-five years. It had been many, many years since I'd seen Margie, admittedly because it might have been too painful. But I'd made it through cancer and chemo. What could rival that?

I told Margie about the pain of Mom not talking to me about her death.

Margie paused, and then replied simply, "Well, I think she thought you were too young. That was the school of thought back then."

Now, having felt for myself the impossibility of being a mother with small children facing death, I was ready to accept such imperfection. It helped that it came from Margie, with a voice very much like my mother's.

The next morning, Margie's ninety-three-year-old husband, Steve, suggested I take home any book of his that interested me. His second floor room was a little dark and as I located the bookcase my focus was pulled to the stereo system and its glowing, red digital light.

The time read 11:11.

I gasped, and my stomach flipped. Tears began falling from my eyes, blue like my mother's, sweet, joyful, tears of amazement and recognition.

Mom, it is you, isn't it?!

I stood still, not wanting to ruin any possibility of contact with my mother. Before my cancer, if anyone had shared this sort of experience, I would have remained skeptical, sure that for myself at least, there was an impassable canyon between me and anyone who had died, much less my mother. But something had smashed all that.

Mom, it's you, isn't it?

I felt a swirl above my head, like the lightest of breezes but different, a pulse that crossed my face and neck, over my repaired breast and around my waist, leaving me with a feeling of being loved so strongly, the essence of me, my spirit, my soul, being loved so, so much.

The most distant of memories, of being held by my mother, rose up to the moment. There was no mistaking it, this love, my mother's hug, though I hadn't felt it for decades.

I also "heard" in a silent voice, "Margie was right. That IS what happened. That's why I didn't say anything. I am so sorry."

My arms hung at my side, my throat aching, my cheeks wet. This was the ultimate emotional gas station for someone who had, in many respects, been running on empty her entire life.

When the swirl began to fade, I looked at the clock again.

11:12.

I said a prayer of thanks and returned to the kitchen where Margie and Steve were sitting at the table. Nothing had happened for them, yet I'd been inextricably changed.

I savored the experience like the most delicious butterscotch candy in my mouth, the sweet flavor of sunshine radiating through me. Still enjoying this secret warmth, I told Steve with a small smile, "Well, I didn't find a book, but thanks anyway."

I found something else. My wonderful, beautiful mother. I had to lose a breast and soldier through cancer treatment to find her, but it was worth it. So, don't be surprised if you see me someday, saddled up next to Ms. Warwick, enthusiastically leading a session of the Psychic Friends Network.

~Patience Moore

45

Balloons

In my family, taking a vacation together was our greater treasure. The four of us would load up the family truck and prepare for the transcendental bliss that came with a lawn chair by a beach. Those trips were the things we looked forward to the most each year, a time for us to reunite without the stress of jobs, school, piano lessons, and dance classes. However, when my mom was diagnosed with breast cancer in the summer of 1999, our vacations went on hold.

Nearly a year later, my mother and I took a trip to Disney World. Because she was still recovering, I had become the adult, responsible for the two of us. I saw to it that her head was covered, that she took her medicine, and that she stayed calm. Our trip to Florida was no vacation for me. While my father was away on business each day, I was to take care of my mother as best as a ten-year-old kid could.

I dragged our bags into our hotel room as I watched my mother scratching her bald scalp under her wig. Ever since she had lost her hair, tension had grown between us. I had come to see her as someone who once was my mom, but who now was this balding woman, weakened by life's sorrows, barely able to hold up the corner of her lips when she smiled. I was not on vacation with my mother. I was on vacation with a ghost.

On our first day, I rented a wheelchair and pushed her around like a child in a stroller. When my arms would start to throb, she would mumble quietly, "Ally, I'm an adult. I can walk." I would push harder, pretending I didn't hear her.

As we entered the park, she saw a man selling balloons and like a child, she requested a specific one, refusing to accept any other then the one she originally wanted. I tied the silky ribbon around her thin wrist. The yellow balloon became a second sun in the sky.

The weather was mild that spring, but regardless, I tucked my mom into the wheelchair with a blanket. She wanted to walk with me, but I still refused to let her. When she wanted to take her wig off, I told her I was embarrassed. I pushed her around from ride to ride, stopping occasionally so she could try and stand, take a pill, eat, or greet a character she loved.

It rained on the second day. As I was preparing our backpack with peanut butter and jelly sandwiches, I heard my mother crying in the next room. I opened her bedroom door quietly. I saw the balloon she had bought the day before, deflated and sagging in the corner next to the bathroom. My mother was sitting on her bed, her feet dangling like the ribbon that held the balloon. Her wig was spinning in her hands and her head gleamed like Mylar in the lamplight. She began crying into the wig.

The door creaked slightly. She looked up at me. I stared awkwardly at the mother I loved and mumbled a question, asking if she was ready to go. She wiped her eyes on the sleeve of her shirt, nodding. I walked over and sat down beside her, my feet dangling like hers off the bed.

"What's wrong?" I mumbled. She nudged her head towards the window.

"It's raining." I looked at the top of her head and noticed the rash that had spread across her scalp. I told her I had an umbrella.

She lifted up the wig to put it on her head. She smiled at me weakly. I could feel the sadness pouring out of her eyes.

As I gazed at my mother, I realized I was ruining our vacation. This was our time to be together, to experience what we had been denied since the cancer had moved in and monopolized our lives.

The day before, my mother had felt alive for the first time in years, and I had stifled her in every way. I had refused to let her heal. We were in "The Happiest Place on Earth," and I wasn't letting her live. I realized that my mother didn't need another doctor. She needed her daughter.

I looked at the floor, ashamed of my behavior, and told my mom she didn't have to wear her wig anymore. She looked up from the window and stared at me in disbelief. I smiled back. She ripped the wig off her head and threw it on the bed. She grabbed a scarf from her suitcase and I helped her tie the knot. In the wheelchair, she reached for the extra blanket. I told her she didn't need it and I packed an extra sweater, just in case.

She soared through the park, smiling at the gray sky, holding my hand, and feeling as alive as the children surrounding her. I bought her another yellow balloon that we tied onto the backpack. She told me she liked that one best.

• • •

I remember my mom was hopeful that day, and not worn down by her cancer. She welcomed whatever would come next, and I was ready to follow her lead. I just wanted her to be happy. With a deep breath, I let her be herself, and watched as she reached for the clouds, embracing life.

~Allyson Hellyer

46

Chicken Soup for the Soul

Love You More

"Goodbye Dad, I love you."

I wait for his usual reply, "love you more," before hearing the click of the dialtone.

"No, you don't," I whisper back.

I am alone in our house, imagining my dad waiting for his plane to take off, his tall legs cramped against the tray table. I'll be sleeping by the time he gets home. I must remember to check in on him when I leave for school tomorrow morning.

A familiar thought pushes its way into my mind. I don't want to consider it but I can't resist. My willpower collapses as I close my eyes and imagine the possibility.

I have to be prepared, I tell myself, just in case.

The phone rings in the dark of night. It can't be time for school already. A few rings later, I realize it's only three 3:00 A.M., and I scramble to grab the receiver before it goes to voicemail.

"Hello," I say groggily.

"Julia, it's Hal. There's been an accident. I'm coming to pick you up. Get dressed."

My pulse momentarily stops as I race down the hall into my father's room. His bed is neatly made, just as he left it two days ago. I hurriedly throw on the clothes lying around my room and frantically wait outside. Hal is one of our closest friends and my dad's business partner. He explains that the plane had to make an emergency landing and some people aboard were hurt. No one knows how badly.

It's the morning of the funeral. I'm in the rabbi's office, flanked by my sister, grandparents and uncles—my father's immediate family. The men from Levine Chapels are here again, handing us our pins of black ripped cloth to wear, to show our mourning. Last time they handed me one, five years ago when my mother died of cancer, I thanked them. They stared at me and replied, "Don't thank us; we shouldn't have to be here." I know better now and just nod as I take the pin.

We enter the sanctuary and silently march in front of everyone to our seats. I was so nervous last time. I started laughing as I paraded down the aisle. I don't want to laugh this time, so I stare at the floor, trying to ignore the sea of black behind me.

At our mom's funeral, my sister read the eulogy. Honestly, I forgot what she said. I couldn't hear her over the hysterical sobs behind me. The whole time I just wanted to turn around and see who the culprit was. Everyone was deeply moved by my sister's words. People talked about it years later. I found a recording and listened to it for the first time, two years after everyone else. It was beautiful. In her smooth, calming voice, my sister read something she'd written our mom that she'd never had the chance to share. How could I compete with that?

I look up and acknowledge the mourners. Sobs are coming from every corner and I try to avoid any eye contact. Taking a deep breath, I start to talk. I hold my composure and never break down. I am a stone. I have to block out the sniffles and loud roars of pain as I read an especially heartfelt passage I had rewritten numerous times the night before. I knew that there must be some combination of words to fit this moment in time; I just had to find it.

We move to the cemetery. This is the worst part. Last time I sat here, my father broke down so hard and violently that his own mother had to hold him in her arms. Now, no one is here *to hold me. I am not listening. I am waiting for the part of the service that has haunted me for five years. They call up the family first to place a shovel of dirt into the hole. Soon, a line will form as everyone contributes a last goodbye. I have to sit here and listen to the nauseating thunk of gravel as it slams into the coffin. I want to yell at them to stop. Please, just stop.*

My eyes flutter open as I come back to reality. No, Dad is not dead. His plane will be fine. It always is. In the morning, he will be home, sleeping, safe and sound. But every time he leaves the house, every time I leave him, I cannot help but think the worst. I tell myself it won't hurt as much if I am ready. Prepared. I have learned to always tell him just how much I love him. To give him hugs repeatedly throughout each day. I will not take his presence for granted. Ever. I have learned that much.

~Julia Singer Katz, age 18

47

How Long?

"You've got a very enlarged prostate that was fine two years ago."

My family doctor's voice changed from his normal friendly yet businesslike tone to something flat and horribly wrong.

"Okay, I've got prostate issues," I thought, trying to look relaxed. "We'll find something to shrink it."

"I'm going to consult a local urologist," he continued. "That way you should be seen next week." By now, his tone was back to businesslike and he was trying to sound casual.

"Uh, excuse me. It's 3:30 on a Friday afternoon," I thought. "What's the rush?"

"I'm also making a lab request for a PSA test. After that you can stop at the Referral Office and arrange an appointment."

It hit me, "Hey, wait a minute, PSA? This isn't funny any more." I wanted to grab my doctor and scream at him to drop the fake, matter-of-fact tone in his voice. I wasn't about to just casually run around with my hair on fire in a clinic for no apparent reason.

WHAT'S GOING ON?

I numbly got the blood drawn. No biggie. Now, just grab the earliest possible date with a urologist and everything's fine.

I said nothing to my wife, Karen. I told myself it was just a false alarm. No sense getting her upset over nothing.

The next morning, my alarm went off and as I was reaching for my glasses, it hit me.

"You have cancer."

Now just wait a minute!

At least let me wake up and get some coffee before I have to digest that!

I made it through Saturday without saying a word, but Sunday night I told Karen I had a urology appointment. We both underplayed it, each for our own reasons.

On Thursday, the PSA results came back. The normal range is zero to four. Mine was twenty-two. They had to be kidding! They must've screwed up the test! I felt fine! Okay. Maybe it was a little tougher going to the bathroom, but I was forty-eight. That stuff happens.

Twenty-two? That's nothing. Watch me whip this thing.

How on earth would I break the news to Karen?

She's a nurse and the initial look on her face said, "Drop the funny guy act right now. My husband is a dead man."

I had just successfully scared the daylights out of my bride. But Karen took the news very well. She was very quiet and calm as we embraced. And then the tears started.

In fact, in that instant, we fell in love all over again. Past disagreements melted away. We knew that tomorrow was no longer guaranteed. Suddenly, the single focus of my thoughts was narrowed down to two words: How Long? Regardless of what else I tried to focus on, it came back. How Long?

With my appointment the next day looming over us, Valentine's Day was different. No joking. Our cards spoke of nothing but love.

A snowstorm had closed much of the town, but our favorite restaurant was still open. Mostly, Karen and I looked at each other across the table and couldn't seem to let go of one another's hands. Each bite was wonderful. Each sip of wine was too. Even the snowfall seemed romantic.

"You have a lump on the right side of your prostate," the doctor said the next day. "I'm sorry. You have cancer."

I shook his hand and thanked him for being honest, but my mind raced.

"Does that mean he's sorry I have cancer, or does that mean, 'You're a dead man, but I don't have the heart to tell you?'" I thought to myself.

"It's very serious," he went on. "But I wouldn't buy any black shrouds just yet."

Whew! I would get a couple of years anyway.

After every visit to the urologist, I made it a point to spoil myself with some momentary pleasure. What did I have to lose?

We spent a magical week on a dive boat in Belize. Normally, cancer would involuntarily enter our conversation every twenty minutes, but by the second day it disappeared completely from our thoughts. We went to Belize to scuba together and we returned refreshed and more in love than ever before.

Thank God for that trip. The reserves of peace and tranquility we built there became essential in our cancer fight. The biopsy numbers were less than cheerful, but I still felt I had a chance. The first PSA reading had been bad. The second one was even worse — thirty-four.

Two weeks later, we were at Walter Reed for screening. Our surgeon examined me, excused himself, and came back with another surgeon, the head of the prostate clinic.

"The head of the bloody clinic?" my mind screamed. "And, why might he be here? I'm a basket case, aren't I?"

An hour later, I was informed that my initial Gleason Score of seven (out of ten) had been changed to eight. That's it. I'm dead.

Forty-five minutes later, as we sat in the group meeting, I started craving a good, strong cup of coffee and something healthy to munch on. I practically ran through the halls of Walter Reed until I found the food shop. I was barely able to keep from pushing people out of my way and almost tore the drink cooler apart, looking for a Frappuccino. I gulped half the bottle down and headed for the register. My nerves were fried. I had to get outside. I spotted a door leading to a patio. It was locked. Just before I started screaming and kicking at the door,

I spotted another one. Biting my knuckles to keep from sobbing out loud, I finally entered the patio, got my breathing slowed down, and returned to the meeting.

• • •

It's been over a year since that day, with one surgery, thirty-six radiation treatments and nine months of hormone-blocking therapy. What a roller coaster of physical setbacks, recovery and internal growth.

I still have cancer. I have no idea what my future holds and I honestly don't care. Today is here, it is special, and I am making it count. I love my wife, my children, and my friends, and I know they love me because we now have the courage to let each other know. Life is good

~Peter Collins

48

Kiss

"Wait here," Audrey tells me. "And don't take your eyes off the luggage."

I do as I'm told, sort of.

I'm a part-time bartender and Audrey's full-time travel buddy and escape agent.

A shinny BMW pulls up, and Audrey, dressed in her finest office gear, waves me in. "Hurry, they may notice before we can get away."

She is puffing on her Gitane cigarette, as any self-respecting French woman would do. "Guy from the car rental gave me keys to this one instead of the piece of crap I paid for."

"And Miss Responsibility didn't give it back?" I ask sarcastically.

"Life is short," Audrey answers, and I notice that my dearest friend is oddly pale.

"I'm blowing off like half of Paris to do this," she says proudly, as we whiz by slower cars.

"Mighty brave of you," I say, knowing that deviating from her agenda makes her frantic.

"I have four doctor appointments tomorrow," she admits.

"Just check-ups, right?" I ask.

"Just some nonsense." She tosses her cigarette out the window.

Antwerp, Belgium, is our destination, because, as per Audrey's request, it's far from Paris, she's going through a Rubens phase, and I want some really good beer.

We rent a room in the cheapest hotel we can find and head outside.

"Museum tomorrow; tonight we get drunk," Audrey says, turning off her phone and heading through the door to a Mexican pub. Before I get a chance to order a Corona, she gets two rounds of tequila.

"One to keep us warm, second to keep us alive," she says.

"We are setting a new record," she adds, and another shot of golden liquid disappears in her red, lipsticked mouth. This is not the Audrey I know, but who am I to argue?

Too many shots to count later, Audrey is singing along to Mexican classics on top of the bar. A group of teenagers are cheering her on, and no one minds that she's making up the words.

"I'm lightheaded," Audrey says, and one of her new fans helps her down to her seat. As she leans forward, her buttondown shirt sags and I notice the all-familiar "X" penciled across her left breast. Audrey looks at me, knowing that now I know. Tears well up in my eyes and as I lean back onto my barstool I miss it by a foot. Everyone is laughing at me and I stay sitting under the table for a good five minutes—stunned.

Four years earlier, Audrey had told me she had cancer the way some announce a change in the garbage pick-up schedule—casually and without emotion.

"I'm going to beat it and we can all get on with our lives. It's a hiccup and nothing more."

I came to see her often. I held her hand and we talked about her kids and my love life without ever mentioning the "C" word. Audrey squeezed chemo sessions in between hair appointments and the piano lessons she had signed up for in order to shorten her "bucket list." Her husband threw her a "Cancer Free" party a year after the initial diagnosis, featuring paintings by an artist obsessed with death. For chuckles, Audrey wore a dress she bought at a boutique specializing in funeral gear.

"You knew I was going to make it, right?" she asked me that night.

"No I didn't," I had admitted, ashamed by my doubt.

I finally stand up and we make our way outside the bar.

● ● ●

"I think my kids will eventually forget me. Not the idea of me, but me, Audrey. Like, that I'm tall and I love chocolate milk and parrots and Rubens."

She bends over into an origami version of herself.

"I doubt it," I say, unknowingly declaring defeat.

A roar, from the deepest part of her belly turns into a frightening, window-shattering scream. I grab Audrey's hand but she pulls away, offended.

"I'm only going to say this once, for all the universe to hear. I'm dying. That is it. And all I really want to do is to live."

A mix of her tears and spit lands on my cheek. I don't dare to wipe it. I hold my breath."You are living," I say.

Audrey grabs me by my scarf and pulls me close. She presses her wet lips against mine, hard. We stay like that, hooked, until she pushes me away. This is not romantic, but the silence it offers is comforting.

"I just want to feel," and she turns around just in time to vomit all over her boots. I hold her hair back just as I have done before. Her confession is over. Audrey looks exhausted.

She no longer acknowledges me. I'm irrelevant. She lights a Gitanes and inhales deeply, eyes closed.

Her fan club from the restaurant spills out onto the street. A drunken teenager steps towards her with a swagger.

"Hey crazy dancer," he says confidently. "Got a cigarette for me?"

"I've got nothing to spare," she replies, without opening her eyes.

~Anetta Nowosielska

Honeydew

The sign on the top of the display case catches my eye.

"Honeydew."

There, in the case, are dozens of beautiful panties in eye-popping colors. This is the brand my cousin had mentioned the night before at her bachelorette party. And there I am, in Nordstrom's lingerie department, with every intention of grabbing a couple more pairs of the generic-brand seamless bikini panties in nude (so they won't show through light-colored shorts).

I think of my underwear drawer at home. Ugh. What a depressing sight. All my undies have faded to a hideous color somewhere between skin-tone and gray. All of them are snagged. But as bad as the undies are, the bras are much worse. I have an inventory of three skin-tone-colored stretchy bras with no underwire, no lace, no support — pure comfort. And three white cotton stretchy bras for walking and doing yoga.

Granted, I have some problems in the chest area. I've had metastatic melanoma in my lymph nodes for over three years. I have two huge scars from two lymph node dissections, one underneath my right arm and the other running above my right collarbone all the way up to my right ear. I have scar tissue around my deltoid, upper trapezius and pectoral muscles from radiation. I have a double port protruding from the left side of my chest. The entire right side of my chest is stained with purplish-black blotches from damage to the lymphatic vessels under my skin. Frankly, I haven't given my nasty underwear much thought, because who cares?

I touch the "Honeydews." Ooooh. They are soft and the lace isn't scratchy at all. A salesgirl swoops in.

"Do you like these?" I ask.

"I LOVE them. They are so cute and so comfortable," she says.

"Hmmm. Do they show through your clothes?"

"Oh no, not at all. They are completely seamless."

Okay. I guess I could believe that. I go for the kicker.

"Do they have to be hand-washed?"

"Nope!" she chirps, "I just use a mesh bag and toss them in the machine!"

Perfect.

The salesgirl helps me find my size in a bunch of fun colors and patterns. Then, I tell her about my bra problem. She seems stumped. How can we find a practical bra that doesn't dig into my skin or have too many hooks or other hardware?

I wander around to the youthful displays at the front of the department. "Hanky Panky" has a cute, light bra with minimal hardware but it's covered in bold stripes and brightly colored lace. I pluck it from the rack anyway.

In the dressing room, I slip on the first pair of "Honeydews."

Oh! They are much smaller than what I am used to and fit like a thong. No way. Then I look in the mirror. Am I really wearing these? They're so pretty and flattering.

Suddenly, I don't feel like a hagged-out almost forty-year-old mom anymore. I can see my abdominal muscles. Perhaps I have more definition around my waist because all the chemo and immunotherapy drugs had sped up my metabolism. Or is it my obsessive-compulsive need for daily exercise? Either way, my abs look good.

I turn around to see what they do for my butt. Magical, those "Honeydews." Even my legs, which are naturally toned, look longer and leaner. By the time I decide to try on the "Hanky Panky" bra I know I am going to love it. Who cares about the bold print showing through my usual uniform of T-shirts? It's adorable and it does a nice job distracting me from the blotches on my chest. I think of my husband, who last saw me in sexy lingerie the day we got married seven years ago. He certainly deserves to look at a "Hanky Panky" bra and "Honeydew" panties. He's the one who has always told me I'm beautiful, in a hospital gown or in flannel pajamas, curled up under a blanket on our faded couch.

Now I see what he sees.

~Gretchen Whiting

50

Chicken Soup
for the Soul

What a Doctor Can and Cannot Do

W hen I was a little boy and sad, my parents would say, "Everything will be better tomorrow. The sun will shine brighter."

As I lay in bed, the night before my wife, Dotty, was about to have a mastectomy, I hoped they were right. I prayed there would be sunshine at the end of this impending ordeal. But I feared we wouldn't emerge unscathed.

I saw myself in the center of a circle, watching cancer patients I had taken care of, and friends and family members stricken with cancer, parading around me. When they stopped circling, standing before me was John, the first patient I had lost to cancer when I was a young intern.

John was twelve years old at the time and like me, he loved baseball. His bedroom was decorated in Dodger blue and white and his souvenir uniform hung next to his autographed Dodger cap.

When I visited him at his house, he was dozing in a fugue-like state. His ghostlike face was covered with large areas of bruising. His skin was shriveled and peeling. He had undergone three unsuccessful courses of chemotherapy. There were no further treatments. John was dying from acute myelogenous leukemia.

My fellow interns suggested the most merciful approach would be to keep him pain-free and let him die in his sleep. But they had not met John. He had not shared with them his dream to see his transplanted Dodgers win the pennant and the World Series.

I gently woke John so that we could watch the last regular season Dodger game. Although I was also a Dodger fan, I professed to being a Yankee loyalist so that I could bond with him. That year, as fate would have it, the Dodgers would be playing the Yankees in the World Series. John's father had died when he was two. I was touched that he had chosen me as his surrogate father, sharing his baseball dreams with me.

"Hey Champ," I kidded. "The Dodgers were lucky to win the pennant. They'll lose to the Yankees in the World Series."

When the Dodgers won the game, John shrieked with happiness.

"I really wanna see my Dodgers beat the pants off your Yankees," he said. "I wanna see them become champions of the world."

I vowed to do everything in my power to keep John alive to see that. I had no more healing skills to offer him. So, the least I could do was indulge him with baseball.

"See you for the series, Champ. We'll watch my Yankees murder your Dodgers."

The next evening, I sat at home, sipping a glass of wine, listening to Beethoven and telling Dotty about John. My first leisurely evening at home in three days was interrupted when the phone rang.

The ward nurse apologized. "Doctor, I know you're not on call, but you left orders to be notified if anything happened to John. He's been admitted in terrible shape. He's pale and sweaty. He's having trouble breathing, grunting with each respiration. He appears to be losing a lot of blood from his G.I. tract."

"Please do a stat hemoglobin and hematocrit and type and cross him for three units of blood," I told the nurse. "I'll be right over, but if anything happens before I arrive, call a code." I remembered the vow I had made.

The blood supply and I reached the ward at the same time. John looked tired and terminal. Unless I gave him the blood rapidly, he would not survive the night. I made a surgical incision into his ankle, attached the blood to a catheter and hand pumped the life-saving fluid into his body. By sunrise, the bleeding had stopped. He was no longer in congestive heart failure.

John opened his eyes and smiled when he saw me.

"Hey, Doc, I hope we're on for the World Series tonight."

We watched all the games in his room, wearing our team caps, drinking Coke, and munching pizza. The Dodgers had won the first three games and we were experiencing the thrill of a potential last game.

"Hey, Champ, my Yankeess will win this game," I kidded, waving the hat I had borrowed from a friend in order to keep up the charade.

"Ain't gonna happen, Doc. The Dodgers will sweep and be world champions."

I must admit that even if I had been a diehard Yankee fan, I would have still been rooting for the Dodgers to win that night.

They clinched the Series. John fell asleep with a smile on his face, secure in the knowledge that his team had won. His dream had been fulfilled.

Several days later, I sat at John's bedside, holding one of his hands while his mother held the other. The priest had just left after administering the last rites. Rain pelted the windows and dark clouds looked like they'd never ease up.

I bid John a silent goodbye. It would be impossibly hard to lose my first patient, but I had learned more from him about courage than I had given him in return. Like his beloved Dodgers, John was a champion. And along the way, I had become a doctor.

Years later, I prayed that Dotty's fate would be different than John's and that there would be more time for us. I hoped the dignity and courage I had learned with John would come to the forefront and that I would be able to share it with her.

When the alarm rang the next morning after a sleepless night, I kissed Dotty and staggered out of bed. It's just beginning, I thought, looking back at her, still sleeping.

"Everything will be better tomorrow. The sun will shine brighter."

~Paul Winick, MD

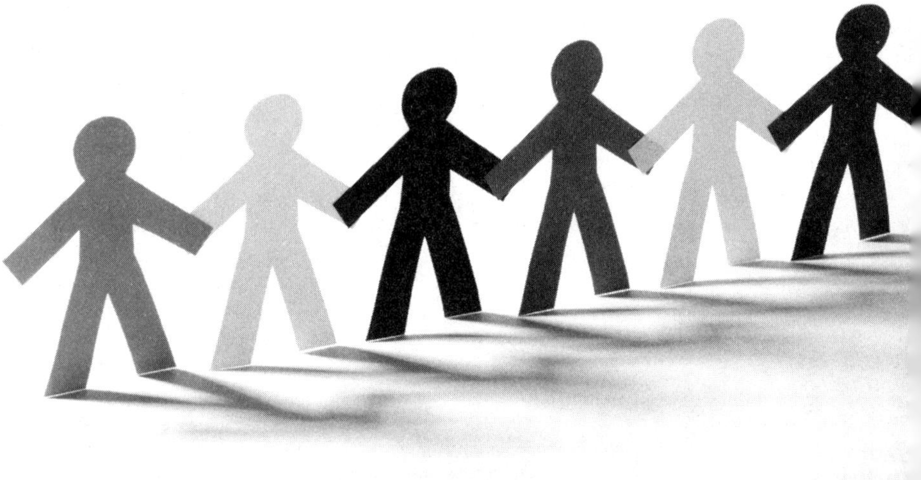

The Cancer Book

Partners

*Lots of people want to ride with you in the limo,
but what you want is someone who will
take the bus with you when the limo breaks down.*

~Oprah Winfrey

51

Chicken Soup
for the Soul

Confessions of a Cancer Caregiver

I am a caregiver who doesn't always love her job.

When my husband, Jim, was diagnosed with lung cancer, I found myself unexpectedly taking care of him. Like many thrust into this situation, I had no prior experience, no medical training, and no proclivity to the position.

I had never taken care of anyone who was seriously ill. I grew up in a home where no one took to his sickbed unless he was near death. Our medicine chest consisted of Mercurochrome, baby aspirin, and a gooey, multi-purpose black salve. We didn't even own a thermometer.

Besides my lack of experience, I am not, by nature, the caregiving type. When we brought our first child home from the hospital, she was colicky and cried most of the time she was awake. Sometimes, at two o'clock in the morning, I would think, "Who is this little stranger interrupting my sleep?"

When our second girl was born, I carried her downstairs, turned on the oven to keep warm (no I didn't put her in it), propped my feet up on the stove, and fed her a bottle while I read a book. I just wasn't one of those mothers who loved to sit and rock a sleeping baby.

So, how was someone with no medical training and no natural tendency for the job going to take care of someone with cancer?

Jim's diagnosis was shocking. He was healthy, had never smoked, and ran five miles a day. Two weeks later, after life-threatening surgery, I was taking home a husband who'd had his chest cut open, a couple of ribs broken and removed, and almost an entire lung excised. I didn't understand a thing about the disease except that it was a very bad one to have. No matter—I was now a caregiver with no instruction book.

At first, my fears weighed me down.

What if I spend the next forty years as a widow?

What if the cancer is growing right now in the other lung?

What if we're living on a pocket of carcinogenic radon gas?

Living with cancer is like living with an uninvited guest in your home. After you recover from the initial shock of his arrival and realize he has decided to stay a while, you must figure out how to adjust. Do you get to know him better so that you're prepared for his next attack? Do you ignore him, and hope he'll disappear as mysteriously as he appeared? Do you make a battle plan?

Soon enough, my type-A personality took over and I dug into my new job with a vengeance. I became determined to do everything humanly possible to save the man I loved.

I had always been a health nut so, in an effort to bolster Jim's immune system, I instigated a menu of holistic remedies.

I tried body brushing, in which the epidermis is sloughed off with a firm brush, using small circular motions, from head to foot. This was a time consuming procedure because Jim has a big body. It produced little, other than a pile of flaky skin and some minor discomfort to an already very uncomfortable patient.

I tried visualization. The patient chooses some sort of scenario that is meaningful to him, like Pacmen gobbling up the cancer cells or a batter slugging the offending cells out of the park. I am sure this works for many people, but Jim just wouldn't play the game.

I tried juice concoctions. Jim consumed so many carrots his hands turned yellow. Adding alfalfa greens didn't go over well, either. When he balked at the nasty tasting mixture, I flew into a rage. "I can't make you better, you know. You have to help yourself."

When Jim finally started chemotherapy, he quipped, "Bring it on, doc. It can't be any worse than what she's been giving me at home!"

At his first session, the nurse described just how I would be giving Jim injections four times weekly to build up his blood counts. She brought me a bag of syringes, cotton swabs, and little bottles of the drugs.

"You should start these at home tomorrow," she said.

"Whoooaaa! Tomorrow? Can't you do it tomorrow and let me watch?"

"Not to worry. Anyone can do this. I'll give you specific written instructions."

"Wait a sec," I said. "Don't I get to practice on an orange or something? The students on ER always get to practice." I could hear the nurse laughing as she walked down the hall.

I am a bit on the obsessive side about doing things by the book. I have no problem with needles or blood, but sticking someone you love in the stomach with a four-inch syringe is unnerving, even for the most stouthearted amateur nurse.

I had Jim lie on a stack of pillows while I assembled the equipment on the table. The makeshift surgery center looked like something out of *M*A*S*H*. I hesitated at every step to ensure I wasn't making some irreparable mistake. God forbid I would lose the patient in his own house.

After about twenty minutes, Jim shouted, "Stick me, for heaven's sake, or I'll do it myself!" Stick him I did, and continued doing so for the ensuing twenty weeks.

With meals to fix and medications to organize and dispense, Jim required around-the-clock care. He needed help to the bathroom and supervision in the shower. I had to clean his surgical wounds, keep his spirits up and his fever down, see that he did his breathing exercises, and answer the telephone.

I must confess, during the first few years when Jim went every three months for scans, I was actually somewhat disappointed when they came back clear! My reaction was troubling. I finally figured out that I would have rather dealt with the cancer than with the fear of the cancer returning. Crazy, I know.

Thankfully, I don't live with that fear any more. Each time a check-up comes around, I thank God that my husband is still here, but we have had to dig deep into our faith to keep the threat of recurrence from robbing us of the joy in his survival.

Jim and I have been living with cancer for six years. While I might not have always loved the caretaker's job, I've always loved the patient.

~Cynthia Siegfried

Our Mantra

There's a thin line between being strong, which is good, and being unfeeling, which is bad. And sometimes, timing is everything—that, and a healthy dose of spirituality.

When my wife, Emily, learned that she had breast cancer, she was at work. Stunned, she called me. I told her I would come over and bring her home.

On my way to pick her up, I was alternately terrified and calm. I wondered how I should react when I saw her. Should I be strong and show no fear so that she could see I was her protector? Or, should I break down sobbing in her arms because I was scared of losing her? I rationalized that I had to keep my cool because I had to drive us home.

As I pulled into the parking lot, Kathie, our friend who worked with Emily, came outside and asked right away, "How are you feeling?"

Her question surprised me. I was waiting to hear how Emily was doing. I started to cry softly. I answered Kathie in fragments. But I dutifully kept my cool.

"Are you ready to go in?" Kathie asked. I nodded.

Emily was deep in shock. When she saw me, she began crying. As we embraced, I let myself cry but forced myself to remain composed.

Later that evening, while Emily was asleep, I sat downstairs at my computer and cried freely. At the time, it was the right decision. The next choice was how to tell our children. It was clear they we had to share the news. We couldn't protect them from something so big.

So, also that first evening, right after dinner, we had our first of four family meetings to share with Carrie, age eleven, and David, seventeen, what we knew. (The other three: three days later when we decided on a double mastectomy with reconstructive surgery; two days later to announce the surgery date; and when the report came in that Emily's lymph nodes were clear.)

We let them know we were scared and that it was okay. But we also assured them we were facing the future with confidence. In order to draw out their feelings, we asked simple questions. "Are you scared?" They were "a little." Carrie noted to Emily, "Your mother had breast cancer and she's okay. Her sister had breast cancer and she's okay. You'll be okay."

Children today have a different understanding of breast cancer than we did growing up in the '50s, '60s, and '70s. Breast cancer used to be a death sentence. Today, more women are surviving. Children can handle the news—and you need them to be part of your recovery team.

Six weeks later, twelve days after Emily's first chemotherapy treatment, I lost my job. Emily was physically and emotionally fragile. In addition, she's the one who had traditionally handled the bill paying, so whenever money became tight she was the first to feel the stress.

I didn't tell her about my unemployment because I didn't want to compound her stress. Only after a trip together to our nutritional oncologist, where I witnessed a new level of strength and confidence on Emily's part, was I willing to take a chance and tell her.

I steeled myself to the possibility that she would panic about us losing the house, and I prepared to condemn myself for hindering her progress by being so self-centered. To my surprise, her response was calm and confident, resigned and spiritual.

"The worst that'll happen is we lose the house, we move to an apartment, and I support us on my salary," she said, adding, "all that matters is that I'm alive."

Once she knew, I could begin to work out a job-hunting strategy, with her in the support role. The role reversal was empowering to us both. In retrospect, I'm glad I waited, but, at the time, holding on to that secret didn't enhance my own wellbeing.

Emily and I were lucky to find a spiritual comfort zone we could share. Meditating and learning about the Kabbalah, the book of Jewish mysticism, opened up many new doors for us.

Individually, we meditated wherever and whenever we chose. Emily favored the backyard in the afternoon. I preferred the bed upon waking and before going to sleep. Together, we meditated two times a week at the chapel in our temple.

We made Love, Kindness, Strength, and Joy our mantra for survival and life.

~Ken Wachsberger

53

Chicken Soup
for the Soul

Freak

People find love when they least expect it. That was certainly true with me. Five months out of liver cancer and a transplant, I was definitely not looking for emotional involvement. Death had been my constant sidekick for over a year. Now it was gone and I was ready to become a reckless college student. I wasn't looking to fall head over heels.

I met Jon and my world changed. What happened next only happens in movies.

When I tried to shake his hand he shouted, "Don't touch me!"

I was thinking, "Freak," when he saw my face and assured me he was sick, not rude.

"Oh, I'm immunosuppressed," I responded. "Thanks for warning me."

In the weirdest moment of my life, Jon replied, "Really? So am I."

It was the most bizarre conversation I have ever had. We exchanged transplant details. Mine was liver; his was bone marrow. He had survived leukemia.

We promised to get together.

I remember thinking, "Something big just happened."

Three weeks passed. I continued my normal life of school and friends. I have no idea what Jon did. Then, I got the phone call that stopped my world. I was having a rejection episode, which is when the body attacks the foreign organ. I was told to get to the hospital immediately.

My friends were incredible. Three of my sorority sisters ran six blocks so I wouldn't have to walk six feet alone. But I wanted someone who understood. So I called Jon. And I remember exactly what I said. "Back in the hospital. Rejection. When does this stop happening?" And in a moment that made my heart leap, he said, "I have a meeting in an hour, but I want to visit you."

I was trying to set up my computer when Jon walked into my room. And right then, my exact thought was "Ooooh, I'm screwed." Because at that moment, I realized that this guy was way more than a crush. We hugged hello and suddenly I started to cry. With my nose dripping all over him, I whispered, "I can't believe I'm back here."

And, while most people would take off if a stranger were sobbing all over them, Jon proceeded to hug me tighter. And he canceled his meeting.

His one free hour turned into three-and-a-half. He asked to compare scars and when I saw his chest covered in them, I melted. We matched. He climbed on my bed and spread his arms around me. We shared stories and told each other stuff we had never told anyone else.

The nurse came in to draw thirty tubes of blood. Jon pulled me on top of him and started rubbing my neck and stroking my hand. Blood was all over the three of us. Jon didn't care. After he left, I'm sure that what I felt was the closest thing to flying that humans can experience.

The nurses asked if he was my boyfriend and when I told them he wasn't, they all replied, "Well, he wants to be."

After years of disappointments, this amazing guy I was head over heels for was liking me back. Maybe I was finally catching a break.

And then, all hell broke loose.

I needed a biopsy the next morning, the same procedure that almost killed me five months earlier.

I woke up and everyone was gone. I told them all to bug off. Jon called and asked how the procedure went. I told him that it didn't because I got too stoned from the meds. I told him it wasn't rescheduled because

I was too scared. I heard him take a deep breath and say, "We gotta talk. I'm coming over." So he came over. For three more hours.

I was still high, and we were cuddling. I decided to risk it, figuring there was more Valium nearby, just in case. So I told Jon I liked him. And what he said next shattered me. I could have handled it if he had said he didn't like me. What he said next has echoed through my head every day since then.

"I would never start something after this."

I felt like I had been hit with a sledgehammer. I guess morphine helps for everything but a broken heart. Jon left, which was normal for a guy who had just heard a girl he doesn't like say how she likes him.

But then he came back for another three hours and continued to hold me because he knew I was scared. And when he left, he said the nicest words anyone has ever said to me. "I know you're scared. Do you want me to come back and stay with you?"

Jon snuck through the ER at 4:30 A.M. so he could sleep on the couch in my room.

We woke up at 10:00. My biopsy was scheduled for 8:00. I freaked out, so he took care of everything. No one ever took care of me. I'm usually the one taking care of everyone else. But at that point in my day, week, life, it was just too many mistakes by too many people.

I had to get out of there. My doctor told me that if I walked out of that hospital, I'd be dead. I didn't care. And then, she said the words that saved my life.

"If Jon were pulling a stunt like this, you would camp out to make sure he did what he needed to do."

Oh my God, that's exactly what he's doing," I said. Point taken. I decided to get my biopsy. I went to check on Jon and found him sleeping on two chairs outside my room.

And guess who stayed with me the rest of the afternoon and cuddled with me because I was scared? Guess who went with me to pre-op and stroked my hand for an hour while I lay there, scared out of my mind? Guess who was sleeping on my couch when I got back and who brought me my favorite drink?

Him.

And guess who's now disappeared from my life?

We had a cancer relationship, I guess. I think about him everyday. I don't know if he thinks about me. I have no idea what happened in that hospital. I guess I'll never know. I'm okay with that. He saved my life.

But I know one thing. Because of Jon, I'm going into pediatric oncology. He made me realize I wasn't alone in the cancer crazy world. I'll devote the rest of my life to doing for others what he did for me.

~Lindsey Goldhagen

54

Chicken Soup for the Soul

A Most Unlikely Partner

come from good teeth. And a Jewish mother. So, when I met George twenty-five years ago on the Upper West Side of Manhattan, I knew right away that I needed to take care of him.

With his shoulder-length shag, Jumpin' Jack Flash bell bottoms, and white Capezio dance shoes held together with duct tape, George was a cross between Steve Winwood and an Afghan hound. Raised by a nomadic family of jazz musicians and left at sixteen to fend for himself, George was camping on the top bunk of a loft rented by a neighborhood wino.

Something like a courtship unfolded. A month later, George moved in, toting a drum, a backpack and a worn down toothbrush I immediately replaced with a blue "his" to join my pink "hers," making us an official couple we married a year later. My wedding gift to him was a trip to the dentist.

I had a mission—motherhood—which we argued about in therapy. George already had two children and reminded me that he barely knew how to be a son, much less a father.

Five summers later, defying logic, I gave birth to Jojo. At the same time, the dentist built a partial bridge across George's uppers. Everybody was smiling!

Jojo and Denture Grip held our marriage together, at least temporarily. But parenthood wasn't a Hallmark experience for either one of us. George could barely push the stroller around without succumbing to a temper tantrum. I felt guilty and trapped, like I was raising two kids.

A few years later, when our marriage had clearly run out of steam, I bought a do-it-yourself divorce kit and filed papers at the courthouse. George rented a shoebox a block away and took Jojo to Vinnie's Pizzeria every night.

George was a hypochondriac. If I had a cold, he had pneumonia. So, when he started kvetching about lower back pain and trouble swallowing, I ignored him. I had enough to keep track of, with three jobs and a growing boy.

Twenty-odd years after we'd first met, George was diagnosed with Stage IV esophageal cancer, already metastasized to the bones. They gave him a year. Although I'd decided long ago that I'd had enough of our marriage, I'd never really had enough of George. I became his primary caregiver and accompanied him for chemo and radiation. I was blown away by the relationships he created with his doctors and nurses. They adored him. They didn't know the George I knew, and I was just getting to know the George they were meeting. Cancer was making him come alive in a new and remarkable way.

I gave George a surprise and bittersweet fifty-second birthday party. He and Jojo went to the movies, their favorite pastime, until George couldn't sit up any longer. By Thanksgiving, the cancer had spread to his liver. By Christmas, it was in his brain. Two months later, George was bedridden, receiving twenty-four hour care from a team of visiting nurses and good friends. I was on autopilot, shuttling back and forth to his studio day and night. He was in horrendous pain, and had it not been for methadone and the Turner Classic Movies channel, I don't know what we would have done.

And then, George's mother showed up. They'd been estranged for years, yet I knew her visit was imminent. She was probably just what George needed in order to let go. He spiraled quickly as she hovered over him, bickering with anyone who came between her and her baby boy.

A few days before George died, I removed his dentures—his mother quickly stashing them into her purse—and proceeded to brush his few remaining teeth. As George lay on his bed, looking at me with a glazed stare, I remembered the day I threatened him with divorce for the first time. It was during one of our therapy sessions, and afterwards, I chose to return home alone, only to find our neighbors hanging out of their windows and looking up from the sidewalk, trailing the flight of Lulu, my very errant dove.

Somehow, she had flown loose, leaving her mate, Kookoo, squawking hysterically on our living room windowsill. People were trying to grab Lulu as she hopped from ledge to ledge, but she was way too quick. This chick wanted out, but she wasn't really willing to go for it. Her final resting place was the top of a cherry tree in the playground next to our building. George arrived home to find me standing there, sobbing.

"Get her," I commanded, pointing up. I had never seen him lift more than a spatula but he scaled that tree as deftly as a monkey and Lulu flapped into his waiting arms. George climbed down the tree to thunderous applause and gave me back my bird.

I noticed a wry smile on his face as he gave a Santa Claus wave to the small crowd before heading back to our apartment. At that moment, leaving our marriage didn't feel like an option.

As I held George and kissed him goodbye, I noticed his snare drum tucked in the corner and a headset perched on his nightstand. He was leaving our life with about as much as he'd arrived with.

George and I were long divorced, but just like Lulu and Kookoo, we were mates for life. Jojo and I, left on the windowsill, would need to find a song to fill the empty space.

~Rosalinde Block

55

What Can I Do to Help?

The exact moment when the news arrived, that cancer had invaded the body of my wife, I knew in my heart that life, as we knew it, would never be the same.

It was surreal. Word spread like wildfire and soon the calls overwhelmed our answering machine.

"What can I do to help?"

This is the most ubiquitous of all questions when it comes to a crisis, so easily and freely asked and yet so difficult to answer at a moment's notice.

The meals started showing up on the porch shortly after the first round of surgery. It was a welcome reprieve after long days at the hospital, and provided a momentary return to some semblance of family normalcy for my two adolescent daughters and me.

Food appeared to be the universal symbol for comfort and help for both those that provided it and for us who received it. In fighting a disease where everyone is rendered confused and helpless, food had truly become the universal means of delivering and receiving nourishment for the body and soul. It almost didn't matter what we needed; the food just kept coming.

Sometimes, more than one meal would be sitting on the porch when we returned home and on those days, the local firehouse became the beneficiary.

Communities of diverse groups of friends, colleagues, neighbors, and congregants had formed naturally to come to our aid. They didn't know of each other's efforts, so coordination and communication became a full-time job for me, negating some of the benefits of everyone's attempts to ease the burden on my family and me. There was no questioning of everyone's motives and good intentions, but for a long time, I struggled to "manage" all of that generosity.

•••

Carole succumbed to her four-year battle with ovarian cancer when she was forty-seven years old. In an attempt to extract some meaning from the total experience, I began to contemplate ideas that would serve to make the caregiving process easier for both the receivers of help, as well as the helpers themselves.

There had to be a simple way to coordinate all the loving efforts of those who so desperately wanted to help, as well as a simple way to be able to accept the help. There needed to be a way to bring all those different "circles of community" together to act as one. There was such a plethora of good information on the Internet aimed at understanding disease, but there were no useful tools that would provide a simple and tangible way to coordinate all these wonderful support efforts.

Thus was born the idea for Lotsa Helping Hands. The basic mission of Lotsa Helping Hands was to create a tool that would be easy to use for all people, be cost-free, and provide a means to meet the burning desire for people to help their friends and family in an acute or crisis situation.

Lotsa Helping Hands has become a web-based service that creates and fosters a community's call to action. The rich, interactive calendar coordinates meals, rides, childcare, and almost any activity that will meet the needs of the family. In addition, features, such as message boards, resource sections, and photo galleries provide a common meeting place for all to unobtrusively keep up-to-date on progress. Although the project started as a cathartic outlet for me to deal with the loss of Carole, it has grown beyond my wildest dreams and is now helping hundreds of thousands of people throughout the country and abroad!

Carole spent her adult life as a nurse practitioner, compassionately helping others through life's difficulties. Although her loss as a wife and mother continues to provide challenges, the inspiration she left behind has been carried on every day that someone finds strength and support through Lotsa Helping Hands. She lived her life with the credo of "what can I do to help?" and now her legacy provides an answer to that question.

For me, it's been a wonderful experience to see how truly giving people can be.

~Barry Katz

56

Chicken Soup for the Soul

The Power to Transform

Two weeks before Christmas, my older sister grabbed our check from the waitress and signaled that dinner was her treat.

"I'm scheduled to have a breast reduction next week and I'm going to need someone to stay with me afterward."

I knew this was her way of asking me to serve as her nursemaid. My sister handled her work and her life as a business and I was a participant in both arenas. Our parents had raised us to always help each other. We were family. That's how it worked.

My sister had provided me with income as a ghostwriter for many of her corporate projects. Negotiation and wheeling-and-dealing were her forte, and I had no qualms about helping her shine from behind-the-scenes. I loved my sister and respected her business savvy, but personally, we were oil and water. She's outgoing, worldly and over-achieving. She's never been afraid to leave the nest, try new things (sometimes fail), and return, ever hopeful and optimistic. In contrast, I'm timid and underachieving, a homebody who has often been sickly.

"I need to feel better about myself," was how my sister explained the surgery. "And my insurance won't cover the procedure after the first of the year."

People like my sister, getting cosmetic surgery, were sending my own insurance premiums soaring. But that was only the first reason why her announcement packed such a wallop. Six years my senior, my sister was inching toward fifty, and while her bosom was always more amply endowed than mine, I suspected that her need to undergo a breast reduction had everything to do with a mid-life crisis. The other antidotes she'd tried to "feel better about herself" included marrying (and divorcing) three times and buying an ocean-front condo in Florida, along with a luxury car.

My sister navigates through her emotional life like a shark. She swallows whatever comes in her path, never fully digests, and has to keep moving in order to survive. I operate more like a crab, crawling laterally through life, slowly mulling over whatever drifts my way. In my thirties, I had battled breast cancer and had subsequently developed heart and kidney trouble. I was convinced that if I'd had a mid-life crisis at all, I was probably anesthetized through it.

"So, what do you think?" my sister asked, slipping her credit card inside the billfold to pay our check. I didn't stop her. Instead, I saw our history reflected in the hazel-colored contact lenses in her eyes. I was her kid sister, the one she had been forced to babysit, the one she had taught how to drive two years after our father died. In the years since, I depended on her, especially during my cancer treatment when I couldn't manage on my own. Yet, as sure as I knew all those facts, I also knew that my sister wasn't asking my opinion any more than she was seeking my approval.

"If it's help you need, I'll be there," I conceded. "I just wish you hadn't chosen right now to schedule this." I explained how I had my own Christmas chaos going on, as well as a freelance deadline. I was ghostwriting an article about holiday anxiety for a local psychiatrist.

"Well, think of it this way," my sister quipped. "Now you'll have direct experience to authenticate that piece for the shrink."

I ended up completing my work before deadline, but it was a struggle channeling the judgments I harbored about my sister's surgery. Repression was exhausting.

With only twenty-four hours before my sister would bid farewell to her God-given cleavage, and I would serve as her nursemaid, I decided to take an afternoon for me. I grabbed my duffel bag and set out for the pool at the YMCA.

As I slipped into my swimsuit, I cringed at the sight of myself in the locker-room mirror. When had I become so bitter and begrudging?

I checked to make sure that Brenda, the name I had given to my false left breast, was properly aligned inside the bra of my bathing suit. Then I flipped on my goggles and plunged into the water.

On my second lap, I spied something bobbing in my lane. I wasn't sure if it was from fog inside my goggles, but I saw the rising arc of a rainbow reflecting out of the water. Muted bands of red, yellow and blue crested over something floating on the surface. Closing in on a now familiar shape, I reached for my left breast as though saluting the flag. When my fingertips met with the flat, sunken ridge of my chest, I realized that Brenda was gone. I sped up my strokes, desperate to rescue her.

At the moment I slipped my renegade breast back into the empty space over my heart, it came to me that I wasn't really peeved at my sister's choice to have that breast reduction, or the timing, or even the cost of my health insurance. No. I realized that plastic surgery could create fairness when life does not. The truth was that a healthy woman of substantial means could buy herself a better body and I couldn't. That was at the root of my feelings—the fact that I just didn't have the power to make things better for myself the same way my sister could.

When I got home, I found a check from the psychiatrist in the mail. I went straight to the bank, cashed it, and invited my sister and some friends for dinner.

"What's the occasion?" my sister asked, when I greeted her later that night.

"Your last supper as a thirty-eight double-D!"

With training bras, in assorted colors, hanging as decorations on my Christmas tree, a small crowd kicked back and feasted on lobster and champagne. It completely wiped out my earnings, but it was worth every penny.

After everyone left, my sister cornered me in the kitchen as I was doing the dishes.

"You know, I really couldn't do this without you."

"Do what?" I asked.

"Any of this—my life." She flung her arms wide as if to catch the world, and her eyes brimmed moist. "I know this must be hard for you."

"Let's not do this." I cut her off, knowing that those few words were enough. I poured out the last of the champagne and lifted my glass.

"To you joining the ranks of the flat-chested."

Our flutes, filled with the bubbly, clinked together. When we took our last sips, I offered up a silent prayer. Mid-life crisis or not, I truly hoped that this surgery would help my sister to finally feel as good about herself as I did about me.

~Kathleen Gerard

57

Chicken Soup
for the Soul

The Front Porch

"I don't think I can do this anymore."

My wife looked at me through huge brown eyes, rapidly filling with tears.

"Yes, you can. You only have five more radiation treatments to go."

I held her close, stroking her hair. She huddled deeper under the covers and relaxed in my arms. Ever since the breast cancer diagnosis, she had tried so hard to be strong. I know she wanted to be strong for the kids and for me.

I had lost my first wife in a car accident and was happy to have taken another chance on love by marrying Becky, my high school sweetheart. When her diagnosis came, my first thought was, there was no way I could go through this again, no way could I lose another wife. Becky knew this. The doctors assured us we had caught the cancer early so we were feeling positive.

We managed to get through her lumpectomy and the recovery from that. After six weeks of radiation, Becky was facing her final five treatments. She was weak, fatigued, and couldn't find her usual fighting spirit. It angered me to see her suffering and burrowing under the covers on a beautiful Labor Day weekend. I felt so helpless and powerless. Once Becky assured me she was okay, I left her to rest.

I went outside. Always one to have a project going, I decided to tackle the front porch. There was wood rot, and some areas that needed to be replaced. As I got outside, long-held frustration and anger erupted in me like a volcano. I took a sledgehammer and suddenly was swinging as hard as I could, pounding and banging on the porch.

I imagined the splintering of wood to be the splintering of my wife's cancer. I couldn't tear the cancer from my wife's body, but I could ravage our front porch, imagining that with every bit of wood I smashed, I was smashing cancer.

With all my might, I pulverized the column that held the porch overhang.

Throughout this whole cancer ordeal, my wife had been very brave. She said she had it easy, because she didn't have to go through chemotherapy.

Looking at Becky today, I don't think it was easy. I felt inadequate at the time because I couldn't fix it. I had to give up control to doctors, surgeons, radiologists, and God. I tried to be strong for her, until that day when she folded and I finally blew.

A while later, I saw her standing at the window, shaking her head. The front porch was gone. I came into the house and walked into our bedroom, not knowing how she would react to the havoc I had wreaked in front of our house.

"Becky, you aren't mad at me, are you?"

She looked at me in surprise. "Mad at you? For what?"

I pointed out the front window. "For tearing down the porch."

She laughed. "Look how sunny this room is now. I love that it's brighter in here."

I was relieved and embraced her, grateful to hear laughter.

"Vince, can I ask you one thing?"

Becky looked at me, still holding on to my hands.

"Sure."

"Why did you tear it down?"

"Well, I couldn't tear the cancer out of you, so I tore down the porch instead."

"Do you feel better?" She asked, crying what seemed to be happy tears.

"Yeah, I think I do." I shrugged my shoulders but grinned at her. "Thanks, honey, for tearing down the porch."

"Huh?"

Becky had a huge smile on her face.

"You comforted me in my darkest hour, Vince, and you found a way to deal with your own frustration. By destroying the porch, you let the sun shine in, and not just into our bedroom."

As I looked around the brightened room that day, I realized the light that filled the space was the light of hope that shines so bright after the darkness.

We never did re-build the porch.

~Vince and Rebecca Yauger

58

Chicken Soup of the Soul

Two Friends' Journey

"Why don't you sit down?"

The doctor greeted me and I obliged.

"I'm very concerned with your MRI."

A sudden sweat came over me.

He went on. "You have a large mass on your shoulder."

What? Could this be cancer? This must be some mistake.

He went on to say that he wanted me to be seen by an orthopedic oncologist.

Oh my God, even he is thinking it might be cancer.

The doctor handed me the phone number of the oncologist, and my body began to tremble, as I feared embarking on the most difficult journey I had ever faced.

I quickly composed myself, put the MRI film under my arm, and headed out the door. Scrambling through my purse, I grabbed my cell phone and dialed my husband's number. I don't think Kevin even knew where I was. Busy getting the kids off to school, I didn't remind him that I was going to the doctor's office today for my results. Between tears and a poor cell phone connection, I managed to tell him the news, and then the call was lost. Hurrying to my car, I called my parents, who live about an hour away. They answered the phone at the same time. I barely managed to tell them the reason for my call when they announced, "We're on our way."

I dialed again.

"Jean, it's me. I just got my MRI results and there's a mass on my shoulder. Can I come over to talk to Mike?" Jean and Mike are my good friends and Mike is an oncologist at Mass General in Boston, the same hospital where my doctor practices. Arriving just a few minutes later, Mike greeted me at the door, wrapping his arms around me in a warm embrace. Taking the film, he headed to his office and closed the door. I went down the hall to see Jean, resting in bed. She has just completed her last round of chemo for breast cancer. We looked at one another and began to cry. Was this really happening? Jean had cancer. Could I have it too?

A few minutes later Mike came in and sat with us. In his calm and comforting bedside manner, one I would come to know well, he explained the tumor. He said it was around my shoulder blade and that it definitely looked like cancer. I leaned over, putting my hands over my face, and cried harder than ever before. Jean held me tight. We might actually be doing this cancer thing together. This wasn't exactly something I wanted to experience with a friend, but I sure didn't want to go through it alone.

Two days later, I whisked my three daughters off to school and headed back to the hospital, with my mom and husband by my side, for more scans and a bone needle biopsy of the tumor. After the biopsy, Mike came by and asked if I'd like the results. I hesitated, but knew I wanted them.

"It's cancer, Pam."

I was diagnosed with Stage III, Synovial Cell Sarcoma. There was no time to waste. My doctors explained that I'd be hospitalized several days at a time for the chemotherapy infusions, with radiation and major surgery added to the mix. With doctor appointments filling up my already busy calendar, I had to quickly get things organized for the unplanned leave of absence I would require over the next several months.

So began my introduction to the angels in my life.

My mom moved in and stayed with us to cover the home front. Jean was feeling better and asked if she could set up a meal chain of friends, just as had been done for her. Friends and family started dropping off dinner for us almost every night and carting our daughters, ages four, ten, and twelve, to their after-school activities. My mother-in-law lived close by and was helping out in every way possible. We felt incredibly blessed to have this circle of support around us.

Arriving at the hospital a few days later for my first round of chemo, I was taken to the room where I would be residing for the next few days. My roommate had her PJs on. Did I have to wear mine? Maybe I could hang out in my clothes for a while.

I was trapped in a room with a view of the Boston skyline and people biking along the Charles River.

I introduce myself to my roommate, Bee, and coincidentally, she was in for a rare shoulder tumor too.

The nurse brought in a scale to get my weight. The chemotherapy "cocktail" has to be measured according to body weight. Okay, maybe I should take my clothes off after all.

A week later, the nausea was gone, radiation was going fine, and my strength had nearly returned. It was great to be home with my family. Chemo was rough and I couldn't help but keep thinking that I would have to go back for more.

I decided to just focus on getting through. It wasn't exactly a walk in the park, but it was a whole lot easier with friends and family jumping in to take care of the day-to-day tasks at home.

• • •

Looking back now, I remember the journey well. Whether it was meals, rides to soccer practice and Girl Scouts, or helping with laundry, friends and family were consistently there.

Jean and I both felt incredibly blessed to have support from family and shared friends during our travels through cancer. Coming together around the dinner table for a warm meal was about the only sense of "normalcy" we could maintain with our families during such a vulnerable time. Our friends were like angels fluttering in with a tasty meal to nourish us. No fanfare, just a kind gesture to warm our hearts and help us through another day. It was quite moving and beyond words. I couldn't thank them enough for reaching out to us that way.

A few months after treatments and with surgeries behind us, Jean and I decided to ask our chain of friends if they'd like to keep the network going in town. The response was unanimous. Thirty-five eager volunteers formed the "Wayland Angels" and set off to help others facing crisis. Within months, families in need were receiving meals, rides, and more. As word of this concept spread, Angel volunteer networks started forming in other communities to provide the same kinds of services.

Six years later, Wayland Angels has several hundred volunteers and has delivered thousands of meals and countless rides for neighbors in need in our community. The Angel volunteer networks are creating limitless opportunity for community outreach, inspiring individuals to establish these partnerships and bring back old-fashioned values of helping neighbors in need.

In today's busy world, small acts of kindness can not only make a significant impact in one person's life, but collectively, these acts can change the entire fabric of a community, reminding us to think of others first, lend a hand to someone in need, and take care of one another.

Facing cancer firsthand, as a family member, or as a friend, is hard. Cancer touches everyone involved. Knowing friends and neighbors are there to help you in your time of need means so much. And, it's even better knowing that someday you can pay that forward.

~Pam Washek

59

Chicken Soup
of the Soul

Salutations

Dearest Patient,

I am one of the oncology nurses who treat you and I would like to offer my perspective of your experience. I'd like to start by commending you on the way you handle yourself through this process. I once had a patient tell me that, "cancer was the best thing that ever happened to me." At the time, I didn't understand her statement. However, through years of observation, I can see that cancer truly brings out the best in many people who make the journey.

You've been through a whirlwind of information and emotions, from the time you first found out you had cancer to the diagnostic process and possibly surgery and/or radiation prior to starting your chemotherapy. Many times, you're not totally recovered from this and you're fatigued and overwhelmed.

When you sit in our treatment area, I wonder what you might be thinking. Are you looking at the other patients and wondering if they have the same cancer? Are you apprehensive about what you are going to encounter? Do you have an idea what to expect? How do you see your process? Do you just want to get it over with, or do you see it as a piece that gets you that much closer to being a cancer survivor?

The one attribute I see in almost every one of you is a desire to survive and do well. Many of you have amazing support systems to help you go through the process. When I first introduce myself and evaluate where you are, I see such courage and strength. As we continue, I usually see you relax and adjust to the schedule and the rigors of your treatment. Again, I am awed by how well you're able to manage your side effects and schedule. I see such willingness to work through your treatment plan. Personalities that like everything in life to be orderly quickly learn to adapt. I sense that no other experience has provoked such a challenge. People who don't initially like to know the specifics of their treatment, or cancer in general, gradually seem to accept and embrace the details. Families who start out focused on getting in and out tend to adjust to the process as well.

I find it equally astounding how much my patients care about me. Often, your first question is how my family or I are doing. It's hard to imagine going through such a difficult process and worrying about someone else before yourself.

Many times I've come to work, my head filled with the trivial problems of day-to-day life and they quickly melt away as I hear about your struggles. I find myself able to give myself to you, if only for the short time we're together. Nowhere else in my life do I see such team work as I see between patients, their families and their health care teams. I feel blessed to be part of it.

I want to let you know what an honor it is to work with oncology patients. I have learned so much from you, from your ability to work through your cancer to your survivorship, all the while maintaining your dignity and sense of humor. I so admire your capacity to be positive and your love of life.

~Sharon Parkes

60

A Love for Listening

Marsha Dale was diagnosed with bilateral breast cancer in 2001. During the enormous struggle of her treatment, including twin lumpectomies, chemotherapy, and radiation, and through the ensuing years of coping with the threats of recurrence, Marsha and her husband, Marc Silver, have discussed every stage of her ordeal.

Or, maybe not. It turns out there is a lot they never explored together and what follows here is an open look at what was once the most popular topic in their household.

Marc: What did you feel when the radiologist said, "Sure looks like cancer to me?"

Marsha: Sheer panic. Disbelief.

Marc: I don't remember what I was thinking.

Marsha: You were thinking, "I can't believe this is happening to me."

Marc: I guess you're right.

Marsha: If it had been you, I'd think, "What am I going to do without you?"

Marc: I was in such deep denial I wouldn't even admit those thoughts.

Marsha: And you didn't come home after I called. You stayed at work. What were you thinking that whole live-long day?

Marc: I just pretended it wasn't happening.

Marsha: You really put it out of your mind?

Marc: I really did.

Marsha: Now I hate you!

Marc: I was afraid to come home because I didn't know what I was supposed to do.

Marsha: You really are selfish.

Marc: I feel really bad about it. I would not do the same thing now.

Marsha: That whole weekend was horrible.

Marc: I took you to a book festival to distract you. That was probably a bad idea.

Marsha: Yeah, it was like, "He thinks he's helping but this isn't at all."

Marc: What could I have done?

Marsha: You could've reassured me, told me we would get through this together. That might've helped. But I was going to be miserable, no matter what.

Marc: It made me feel so bad that I couldn't cheer you up.

Marsha: But you thought, "Oh, I'll just get her mind off it." That's a typical guy thing.

Marc: I had a bad track record as a cheerleader. When one surgeon recommended a double mastectomy, I said, "I won't mind. I'll love you without your breasts!" I thought that would make you feel better.

Marsha: And I said, "How would you feel if they were going to cut off your penis?" Did that upset you?

Marc: Well, I tried not to take it personally. I was just stunned by how deeply affected you were. It's hard for a guy to understand.

Marsha: When it started to get very real and I thought about having no breasts, it freaked me out.

Marc: Even with reconstruction?

Marsha: I knew I wouldn't get sexual pleasure from reconstructed breasts. It was a gut reaction.

Marc: A week after your first chemo, we went to the wig shop.

Your hair was starting to fall out and you were crying a little. I asked you to try on a goofy wig. Was I out of my mind?

Marsha: Usually I'd say, "Cut that out." But I figured, "Why not?" And we laughed. I hadn't laughed like that in two months. That was a day I really dreaded, but laughing at those wigs took the sting away.

Marc: In those first weeks, did you ever think about sex, like, no sex for the next nine months?

Marsha: No sex because I'll be bald and unattractive and who would want sex with me?

Marc: But we did.

Marsha: We did.

Marc: You were nervous about me seeing you without your wig. But I saw you all the time like that.

Marsha: But not in a romantic situation.

Marc: You have a very pretty head. It's elegant and sleek, kind of like a space alien!

Marsha: Did you ever think I might die?

Marc: When the doctors thought they found lymphoma, I thought, "This is it. Cancer is going to destroy us." But I never told you how scared I was. I cried in the car and I never told you.

Marsha: What was I going to do if my husband freaked out? It's a good thing you didn't tell me!

Marc: One thing that kept me from freaking out was seeing your courage. You dealt with all those awful treatments with such dignity and grace. I don't think I could have been as strong.

Marsha: If you had said to me, "You're going to get breast cancer and it's going to be bilateral," believe me, I would have said there's no way I could handle it. But this taught me something: Whatever you think you can't handle, when push comes to shove, you can. How did you cope?

Marc: It helped when I'd take a bike ride or a run or a yoga class. Did you mind when I did those things?

Marsha: No, I knew it was important to you. I never really resented it.

Marc: I can't even begin to tell you how much it helped to get a break from cancer. Another thing that helped were what I called "limbo days," when we were waiting for test results. I was so happy, because for a few days, nothing could happen. We could just order Chinese food and watch TV. Like normal.

Marsha: I was the opposite. Waiting for news, my thoughts were never happy. You can call it pessimism. The way I term it is, "I'm a hard-core realist."

Marc: Didn't you want to hope that everything would be okay?

Marsha: Every time I would think that, I would think of the Jews in Nazi Germany. They'd think that it couldn't get worse, and it did. I wanted to think, "I'm going to rise above cancer." But in my dark moments, I'd say, "Who am I kidding?"

Marc: You're a pessimist and I'm an optimist. I realized I could be me and you could be you, and it's okay. That realization didn't weaken our marriage.

Marsha: You didn't think it was a major disappointment that I wasn't more optimistic? Even now, when I sound negative and you're like, "You shouldn't be negative," it pisses me off. I wonder, is that chipping away at our relationship?

Marc: Sure, sometimes I'd think, "Why can't she be like me?" But people are very complicated, and it would be stupid for me to expect you to be exactly like me.

Marsha: What really helped me get out of my negative thoughts is that I have one life. This is it. We don't have a next life, unless you're Shirley MacLaine. It makes me think I should live the best life I can and to enjoy it as much as possible.

Marc: Easier said than done!

Marsha: You think cancer changed our marriage?

Marc: I do. Our relationship is deeper. We've been through a war. I hate to use that cliché, but it really is like going into battle and fighting this enemy. If you can stay together and fight it, it strengthens you. I hope I was there for you, even if we weren't always in the same place. Do you ever wish you'd had a different husband to go through this with you?

Marsha: No, because I can't imagine another person doing what you did for me.

Marc: What did I do?

Marsha: You were just there. And you did what you could. You put everything aside and took off from work and sat in doctors' offices and took notes. You made funny comments and made me laugh, like when we came home at midnight after spending six hours at an emergency room to find out what was making me short of breath, and you said, "Honey, you can't say I never take you anywhere!"

Marc: I have a great team of writers.

Marsha: You shouldn't get a swelled head, but I do say, "Thank God I have a husband who was there for me."

Marc: You still love me?

Marsha: I do. Do you still love me?

Marc: I do. You're very special, even if you are a pessimist!

Marsha: Sometimes I wish you were more romantic, that you'd hold my head in your hands. But your ability to make me laugh got me through. You want to talk about chicken soup for the soul? That was the chicken soup, even more than when you made me a meal.

Marc: I'm going to take your advice and hold your head in my hands and give you a kiss.

~Marsha Dale and Marc Silver

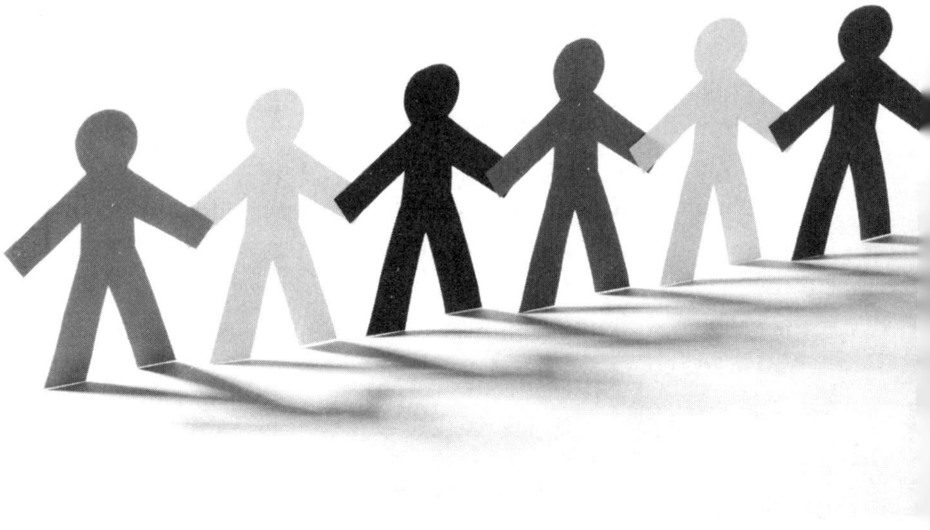

Chapter 7

The Cancer Book

Loss

Life is a shipwreck but we must not forget to sing in the lifeboats.

~Voltaire

Chicken Soup
for the Soul

A Promise to Keep

As a child, Melissa always had her very own nighttime ritual: brushing her teeth, washing her hands and face, putting on PJs, and snuggling in bed. Before drifting off to sleep, she liked me to rub her back, sing "Puff the Magic Dragon" and talk about the day.

All too quickly, her childhood routine was history, as my little girl grew into a beautiful young woman, ready to make her mark in the world. It had been years since I sang her to sleep.

Yet, there I was, my daughter once again curled in my arms, singing of magic dragons which never die, in faraway places where the sun always shines. Since Melissa had been sick, this part of the old routine, long abandoned along with baby dolls and make-believe ponies, had once again defined our nightly ritual. Though no longer a little girl, Melissa folded into my embrace like so many years ago, safe and secure, unafraid of the darkness that filled the room.

I was fairly certain that it wouldn't be long. For two difficult years of chemotherapy, radiation, a bone marrow transplant, and experimental drug treatment, Melissa had exhibited dignity and grace, always living even when she knew she was dying.

She interrupted my song.

"If you have learned anything from me through all of this, make sure you use it," she whispered, seemingly ready to take her next—and final—step.

I told her I was proud of how she had lived her life and that I had learned many important lessons from her.

"Everyone says that to me," she sighed, weakened by the advanced stage of her disease, "but I'm not sure that everyone will really do anything differently because of it. Promise me you will do something to make a difference, to make things better."

"I promise," I said.

•••

Melissa died three nights later. She was nineteen years old.

Nothing can prepare you for the death of your child. No matter how much time you think you have to get used to the idea, the pain cuts deeper than any heartache you've ever imagined.

What should I do? Would she still hear my song about a dragon by the sea? My world had turned upside down and I needed to make some sense of it all.

We had agreed to bury Melissa's ashes in a new garden that we would build in her honor, just as she'd asked. Preparing her garden gave my life short-term purpose in those sad days right after she died. While I dug sod and raked rocks in our weedy side lawn, the July sun burned as brightly as her spirit, guiding each turn of my spade.

I had time to reflect on her last request, to figure out how to keep my promise. With every shovelful, I pondered, "What have I learned and what will I do with it?"

Slowly, my daughter's lessons became clear.

Live each day with purpose. Focus on what's really important. Value the friendship of others. Advocate for what you know is right. Keep your dreams alive. Seize every opportunity to be creative. Be grateful for gifts received. Never give up hope. Cherish each moment.

In her own short life, Melissa had lived each day exemplifying these simple but profound truths. I needed to find a way to use what I had learned from her. An idea began taking shape along with her garden.

I had seen firsthand the effects of a cancer diagnosis on a teen-ager, and watched as Melissa tried to navigate a health care system not designed for adolescents. Though Melissa was no longer a child, she hadn't yet experienced life as an adult. She was only seventeen years old when she was first diagnosed.

Just as she was preparing to venture into the world, her plans were interrupted. Instead of going to the Ivy League university to which she had just been accepted, Melissa found herself in the pediatric oncology clinic of our local children's hospital, sitting on chairs too small and staring at paintings of circus animals, with nothing to read but *Highlights for Children*. As her disease progressed and she began experimental drug treatment at an adult cancer center, the surroundings were even less appropriate for this vibrant young girl who still believed her emerging dreams would come true.

After watching four children become teenagers, I had grown accustomed to the normal angst of adolescence, but it all paled in comparison to the suffering of being a teenager, like Melissa, with cancer. Wasn't it enough that she was bald, pale, and physically exhausted? It just wasn't fair that she should be home with her parents on a Saturday night, instead of having fun with her friends at an all-night concert. There were absolutely no support systems in place that could help her feel normal.

As Melissa's garden grew, so did my plan to find a way to support other teens who were falling through the cracks. Ten months after she died, I established Melissa's Living Legacy Teen Cancer Foundation with the hope of keeping my promise "to make a difference — to make things better." Thanks to Melissa, we're doing just that.

Eight years later, time hasn't dulled the pain of missing her but I can now smile through my tears and be grateful for the gift of this incredible girl who inspires me to live each day with purpose, mindful of simple joys and small blessings.

Every morning, before I sip my coffee from the delicate china cup she gave me, I walk outside into her garden, thankful for all I've been given. I ask God to protect my family and to keep my daughter's spirit alive. I pray for the strength to make at least a small difference, so that when I see my girl again, she'll welcome me home and say, "Good job, Mom."

~Lauren Spiker

62

Evelyn's Story

E velyn first came to see me eleven years ago because of a groin node. She was pleasant, well groomed, and elicited admiration and empathy. While examining her, I ran a quick mental tally: a groin node might signify infection or lymphoma. Most seriously, it could mean cancer.

The node's appearance told me very little. We hoped it was benign, and if not, that the malignancy would be amenable to therapy.

Personally, I found myself wishing for anything that was best for Evelyn, even if that included the most unscientific kind of miracle. But as a doctor, I must invariably guard my inner feelings from my patients.

My heart sank when I saw the pathology report. Evelyn had ovarian cancer. Hopes and wishes, the currency I had traded in, precipitously lost their value.

When we met ten days later, I felt my professional shield take its place, putting forth a neutral position that could almost be interpreted as indifference. We adopt this posture at times in order to save ourselves from being blown away by a tornado of emotion. This is particularly true in the face of a cancer diagnosis, especially one that might mean death in a matter of weeks or months.

I often tell patients that, as a surgeon, I don't necessarily know the latest literature, newest chemotherapy or other therapeutic modalities and certainly not the prognosis. I do this to avoid any confusion and misplaced dependence.

It's more truthful to tell a patient, "Your oncologist knows best."

That's what I told Evelyn. I wasn't sure at the time if she could feel the despondency and pain weighing down my words and slowing my speech. In that moment, I was more than a scientist; I was a priest, a witch doctor, a shaman in a white coat, but all in all, I was powerless.

Evelyn's disease had spread beyond the confines of her ovaries and pelvis. It had already invaded her lymphatic and venous systems. It doomed her to death.

And yet, she was nonplussed.

"I have ovarian cancer in my lymph nodes," she said, repeating my words.

I nodded.

"I am a goner. No?"

She smiled. There was no sense of doom and no cries of "why me?" in her eyes. Most people with a severely advanced disease like hers were usually heartbroken and bitter.

The oncologist called to communicate her opinion. Evelyn was unlikely to survive more than a few months. That confirmed my own opinion. Because I had retracted to my physician's crouch, I pretended I felt nothing. But like a turtle, I tapped on my shell and felt the hollowness of my conviction. I cared. I shed invisible tears. I worried about the pain that would accompany Evelyn in her last days.

The logic of cancer, or the total lack of it, required that I forget Evelyn. I lived a life of the living and was not going to waste inordinate amounts of time, energy, and passion for someone bound to die. My energy and passion was for the living. Evelyn's next stop was Death.

In most cancer stories, Evelyn's would end right here. But she wouldn't die. She went along pleasantly, with an inner sense of tranquility and a mysterious satisfaction with her daily life. She had an unspoken faith and never questioned why she'd been stricken with cancer.

Her oncologist and I talked about her often. As the years passed, her wonderment seemed to be expressed in the changing, increasingly incredulous pitch of her voice. Evelyn was her most lasting success, she said, in an ever-expanding cascade of words. She was a phenomenon, which, time and again, words failed to adequately describe.

Evelyn defied all logic. She had literally beaten a brand of cancer that had felled many stronger women. Naturally, the medical world around Evelyn attempted to decipher if she was a genetic freak. In the end, nothing distinguished her from other ovarian cancer sufferers.

Evelyn reminds us that our diagnostic arrogance is sometimes inappropriate and not always based upon any real certainty. There is always that chance that someone will escape the suffocating walls of prognosticators. My oncology friend sounded like a proud parent recounting a growing baby's progress. She was an important reminder that hope was not an empty vessel.

Hope was fueled arbitrarily and continually, with new scientific discoveries, new chemotherapeutic agents, and new therapeutic combinations. As the scientific tool-kit expanded in Evelyn's care, the time between diagnosis and her demise was extended. I saw her at intervals and wondered about her survival.

You can never tell when a new drug will arrive and melt your disease away. This was the lesson I learned as I saw Evelyn, time and time again.

But hope must be buttressed with solid pillars. As a scientist, I affected a clinical neutrality while the human me cheered her on. I wanted Evelyn to live forever.

After eleven years, she couldn't take any more chemotherapy. Life had become too much of an aching burden. She passed away quietly, grateful she'd seen many more summers and springs.

Evelyn's life reiterated a few things about cancer: that in addition to being a pathology, having cancer was also a way of being. Evelyn accepted it and lived with it, at peace, without complaint. As each malignancy is different, so is every patient different from all others.

Evelyn found a way of living that was hers alone. I tell all my patients to find a way to live with their cancer. To me, that was Evelyn's lesson.

~Pius Kamau, MD

63

Chicken Soup for the Soul

Three Weeks of Silence

As I was being pushed to the operating room, I tried to relax, as much as anyone could under those circumstances. I'd done this before so I knew the drill.

Squamous cell carcinoma in my throat.

Eight years ago on the left side, now on the right side. I'd be good as new after the operation, chemo, and radiation. Just like before.

Except when I woke up it was different.

My husband, Richard, stood next to me with an anxious look in his eyes.

"You've got a tube in your throat," he said. "The doctor found that part of the cancer was on your larynx and he had to scrape pretty hard to get it off. The tube needs to stay in until your larynx is healed."

"Oh," I tried to say. "How long will that be?"

Nothing came out. I put my hand to my throat and, sure enough, a tube was sticking out. At least I wasn't in much pain. Looking at Richard, I pointed to my throat, then my mouth, and somewhat sorrowfully shook my head to indicate "No."

Richard patted my hand and said, "It'll be okay."

That was my first effort to communicate without a voice.

When I came home, my friends Sue and Nancylee were the first to welcome me. Sue brought some delicious rice pudding and Nancylee brought some special soup made from a secret family recipe. She told me that soup was all she ate for six weeks after her lung cancer operation and it had saved her life.

I tried to communicate my thanks, but she stopped me gently.

"I brought you something else, too," she said. "You won't be able to talk to Richard for a while, so I made you this sign. Here's everything you need to tell him."

She brought out a piece of cardboard about the size of two sheets of paper, divided into four sections: "Yes," "No," "I Want a Drink" and "Get Lost."

We howled with laughter as only good friends can. When we calmed down, Sue said, "The sign will work fine if he's in the room, but you need a way to call him if you can't get out of bed." She ran out of the room and came back with a crystal bell.

"You can ring this if you need him. Now, you're all set."

By this time I was getting tired, so Sue and Nancylee left, secure in the knowledge that they had provided me with the means to communicate until I regained my voice.

As it turned out, I didn't use the bell or the signs very much. Richard turned out to be an unbelievably perceptive caregiver. The first night I was home, I thought fleetingly that he might move to another room so he didn't have to hear me coughing all night. (The tube caused a lot of coughing and hacking as my body produced copious amounts of mucus to rid itself of what it considered an intruder in my body, much like the body tries to reject a transplanted organ.)

I don't believe it ever crossed his mind. He slept next to me, as he had for fifty-one years, and woke up immediately at any sound I made, no matter how small. I was reminded of the instinct a new mother acquires that enables her to wake up immediately when her baby stirs—an instinct that comes from love.

During the daytime, I had plenty of time to reflect about the communication between us. Much of it was gestures and facial expression, but we wrote a lot of notes, too. I had to improve my handwriting a bit to make that process work, but writing out everything is cumbersome, so I thought carefully before trying to communicate.

Many times I realized that what I wanted to say was going to be something negative like, "Why can't you ever pick up your socks?" Since I couldn't talk, I didn't say it, and I realized that perhaps too much of my previous communication might have been negative. I vowed to try and change that when I got my voice back.

I also realized that because my facial expression was a major means of communication, I might want to smile a bit more. Richard took great care of me. He made me milkshakes when I didn't feel like eating, cooked when I did feel like eating, and took care of all the household details. I wanted to show him that I appreciated everything he did, but I am by nature a rather serious person and don't smile a lot. I made a conscious effort to smile more so that he could tell I was pleased and happy.

Three weeks after the surgery, we went back to the surgeon's office for follow-up. I was convinced that the tube could be taken out, and disappointed when he told me that it would have to stay in longer. Richard once again read my mind and asked the crucial question.

"What are the criteria for removal?"

"She has to be able to talk and to breathe on her own," my doctor replied.

When he stepped out of the room, I looked at Richard, put my finger on the tube to cover the opening, and said my first words.

"I can talk!"

But it wasn't enough. I still couldn't breathe with the tube covered.

That was three months ago. In a few weeks, we will go back to the doctor, again in the hope that the tube can be removed. This time, I'll go back talking fluently and also being able to breathe with the tube closed. I think I've had this tube long enough to have learned the lessons it had for me.

"Think before you talk" has become a reality rather than just an old proverb.

~Eleanor Bergholz

The Shower

Warm water probes my bald head,
where long hair used to diffuse
the chains of drops.

Savoring a moment of being alone,
I glance down to watch the water
leave my feet and run to the exit.

Strangely,
I see a clear view
of only one foot.

The other,
partly obstructed
by the intrusion of my breast.

Ah, yes.
Cancer.

~Laura L. Strebel

The Healing Power of Ice Cream

As with many sons in my generation, my father and I were not as close as we could have been, but when I made my decision to follow his lead by joining the Air Force he was excited and happy. I became an aviator and now lead a squadron on the beautiful island of Guam.

During the first part of my tour in January 2006, I received a life-changing call from my father. We discussed his illness, diagnosed as kidney cancer, and how he would combat the six-month prognosis he'd been given for survival.

Initially, I believed he could overcome this hurdle, while also knowing that my optimism might not be enough to ensure success. I told him I loved him and gave him the only advice I could come up with.

"Dad, it may not seem like it, but you have been given a gift. You now know when your time is coming to an end so you have the chance to fix the things that need to be taken care of."

A few months later, I returned to Kentucky for a visit. My father's kidney had been removed and he was doing chemotherapy three times a week. After the horror stories I had heard from other cancer patients, it wasn't anything like what I had expected. I was amazed at how easily he took to the entire procedure. He made friends with other patients and the nurses attending him. I was shocked to see him eating cookies and napping. He even asked me to go out and eat with him afterwards. I returned to my base, more convinced than ever that my father would beat this disease.

That Christmas was the first in many years where both my sister and I were home to visit our parents together. Even though my dad had lost a great amount of weight he looked good and had already outlived his original prognosis of six months. I looked forward to seeing him in the spring when I returned to the States for training.

As fate would have it, I was able to spend my forty-fourth birthday with my father before returning to Guam. During that time we talked and visited with his doctor. I was disheartened to hear the illness was back and spreading quickly. His time was short, no matter what procedures were tried and he needed to make a decision on what course of action to take.

Those four days were tough. While looking at property for me to purchase as I near the end of my military career, we stopped at the local Dairy Queen to have lunch. As a child, I had seen my father always eat his ice cream in a bowl. But on that day, he ate an ice cream bar for lunch and then decided that it was so good he needed another, and then a third one for the road.

Early the following morning, as I was packing my car to begin my trek home halfway around the world, my dad told me he was discontinuing his treatment. I was extremely hurt. I couldn't bring myself to talk much and shortly thereafter I left for the Louisville airport.

A half mile down the road I remembered my mother's saying about unspoken words and I realized there would be no more ice cream lunches. I went right back to the house and stepped up on the porch where my dad was sitting in the dark, reflecting on his life, I suppose. I told him I loved him and I would miss him. I let him know I was never disappointed in him. I believed in him because he was my dad!

Three weeks later, I received a call from his doctor, a former military officer who always kept me updated. My father was in the hospital and I needed to hurry. The Air Force was great to me and got me home quickly, joining my mother and sister at my dad's bedside. Eleven hours later, he died.

In that brief time, I realized many things.

His initial decision to forego further treatment, which I did not agree with at the time, had been correct. He'd been in severe pain. His nurses told me that he had fought to stay alive just to see me one last time. Even though he could no longer speak when I arrived, he did recognize me with a hand squeeze and uttered a simple "hey buddy." That was my gift.

During the funeral, many people told me about my dad coming to visit them. He had taken my advice and actually visited all his friends and made amends or regenerated old friendships. He made things right, not only with his earthly relationships, but also with God.

Ice cream now takes on a new meaning for me. When things are tough at work and I only have time for a snack, sometimes I just grab an ice cream bar. It brings me peace and keeps me grounded, while helping me remember a man who endured a lot of pain just to say goodbye to his son. I miss you, Dad!

~Joe Hayslett, Jr.

66

My Regret

"Erika, go get me a beer!"

I looked at my mom with her bald head, blotchy skin, open pus-filled sores on her lips, and IVs and catheters.

"Psst, Erika! Make it a cold one," she added, using her "don't defy me, I'm your mother" voice.

"I can't, Mom. It might interfere with your meds."

She plopped back on her pillow, defeated, and wouldn't look at me.

Mom was dead a few days later.

• • •

It's been twenty-two years.

What I remember most from those last days and my mom's battle with lymphoma is that unfilled request.

Mom was a fighter. She always had a "can do" personality, and if anyone could lick something by putting one's mind to it, it was my indomitable mother. But even though she tried, she couldn't lick cancer.

Mom was diagnosed when she was fifty-nine. She finally consented to see a family doctor after finding she had no energy to climb her driveway. He suggested hospitalization and running tests. She pooh-poohed his recommendations.

Within a couple of weeks, I found her lying on the couch with labored breath. I'd brought my infant son up to New Jersey from North Carolina to see Mom. Her neighbor took care of my baby as I drove Mom to the hospital; Dad was out of town on a business trip.

Mom was very weak, and we were initially left languishing in the emergency room waiting area. I told the very passive clerk that I had heard a death rattle as Mom slept. I knew the sound because I'd heard it before when my grandma went into heart failure. The clerk paid me no mind. I called my husband, who was an internist back home in North Carolina.

"Tell the clerk your mother is a GI Bleeder," he advised. "That'll get her seen."

I did just that. Abracadabra. Open Sesame! Those were the magic words!

Mom was wheeled in. Within a couple of days, we knew she had lymphoma. The oncologists were positive that if she would follow a regimen of pills and follow-up spinal taps she'd live another eight to twenty years.

Mom eventually resumed teaching, which was a stressful job, but she wanted the health insurance coverage and the retirement benefits. A year later, I had another boy and my sister had a girl. Mom enjoyed being a grandma.

Two years later, Mom retired. She spent a year going on sundry trips to Arizona, Costa Rica, and South America. She entertained guests from England and Japan. The final year of her life, my mother accompanied Dad to the Far East for a month long business trip.

Shortly after my third son was born, Mom went into the hospital. Her cancer had returned with a vengeance. She began massive chemotherapy. Her hair fell out in clumps.

I flew up with my infant son. The doc said Mom was not responding. I fled the hospital and secluded myself in my parents' bathroom and howled in the shower.

I called my husband. He began contacting physicians at Duke and U.N.C. who might try some experimental drugs to enable Mom to have a bone marrow transplant. Hope again.

Mom was glad to go to Duke, full of sweet memories of her alma mater. She was a Yankee who had fallen in love with the South during her days at Duke. She instilled that love for North Carolina in me.

In the remaining weeks, when the kind physicians tried to get her healthy enough for a bone marrow transplant, I visited Mom each day with my nursing infant. I handed off the babe to Dad in the lobby, while Mom and I sat and talked in her room. She'd look out her door at the hairless children strolling the hallways with their parents.

"I am so lucky I never had to go through what those parents are dealing with," she said with watery eyes. "It's bad enough for an old woman like me to endure this dreadful disease, but it's just cruel for those innocent kids."

• • •

Days before Mom died, she said, "Erika, I want to die."

"No, Mom. No, you don't want to die. You must work with the physical therapist to get stronger. You'll get better."

She shook her head. "Sweetheart, I want to die. Let me go."

"No, Mom, you have so much more to look forward to."

A tear formed in her eye, and she closed them. I sat there while she napped. When she awoke, she looked around, startled.

"What's wrong, Mom?"

"Oh, I had the best dream. I was a little girl on my grandpa's farm in Pleasantdale."

Mom fell into a coma that night and died a couple of days later. She was buried in Pleasantdale Cemetery, next to her parents, near her grandparents and great aunts, and close by her great-grandparents.

On her stone is written "Be Gentle with yourself. You are a Child of the Universe."

Having cancer gave Mom time to recognize her mortality and to appreciate each day she had, and to live each one to the fullest.

I have regrets. I'm sure most children do when struggling with a parent's illness. One of my biggest is that I didn't listen to Mom when she made a request of me. Instead, I followed the rules. If I were to do it again, and my mommy asked me for a beer on her deathbed, I'd sneak one past the nurses' station for her, and one for me too. We'd sip those cold brews with one hand on a can while our other hands held tightly to each other.

~Erika Vogel Hoffman

67

The Letter

There sat my father's small black duffle bag, made of rugged, now worn, nylon with his name, David C. Bodell, stitched in white across the top flap. It was his case for the essential items he always carried with him: his pipe and tobacco, pilot log book and company badge, pictures of his wife and three children, calculator, keys to the house and dock where he kept the sailboat, sunglasses, driver's license, credit cards and money. He never went anywhere without it.

Dave, as he preferred to be called, was a true pilot—he received his pilot's license even before his driver's license. He flew professionally, first for Pan American crisscrossing the world, and subsequently for United Airlines on the mighty Boeing 747-400, between Los Angeles and Australia, enjoying warm weather no matter the season.

At the age of fifty-five, Dad was diagnosed with late-stage prostate cancer. Although company policy requires all pilots to undergo annual physicals, including prostate exams, the malignant tumor grew on the opposite wall of the gland, where it could not be physically examined.

By the time symptoms compelled him to see a doctor, he was Stage IV. Recommended surgery meant removal of the prostate, along with extensive chemotherapy and radiation, which could prolong his life, but would almost certainly leave him severely debilitated.

A man of extraordinary pride and intellect and intensely devoted to his family, my father opted for a hormone treatment, shrinking the prostate and slowing the inevitable spread of cancer. He had asked his doctors to facilitate a "life of quality, not quantity." This decision was undoubtedly for his family, maximizing the quality time we would enjoy with him without putting us through the emotional pain and experience of witnessing his physical and mental deterioration. This was his selfless character.

Over the next year-and-a-half, Dad was active and symptom-free, and, without any visible degeneration, it became easy for me to ignore the fact that the disease even existed. That is, until a certain event changed my perception.

As a son of an active pilot, I received discounted airfare, which I often enjoyed. During the summer between my sophomore and junior years of college I planned a trip to Singapore. One of my closest friends, who had recently lost her father to lung cancer, offered to take me to the airport. At the gate, she gave me a hug and handed me a gift bag containing magazines, candy, and a card, which she asked me to read once I was airborne.

Seated comfortably on the upper deck of a 747-400, I requested a glass of wine and opened the card. Her message was simple enough—your father is dying and you have not accepted it.

She was right, of course. I had spent plenty of time with my father, shuttling between college and home, living the same lifestyle we'd had before his diagnosis. But I had not addressed with him the inexorable ending his cancer would bring, nor had I acted on the precious opportunity, while he was still alive, to tell him exactly how I felt.

Somewhere around 33,000 feet this epiphany occurred, and I asked the flight attendant for some paper and a pen. She returned with the airline's stationery and another glass of wine and I began writing the most important letter of my life.

The letter laid out, in the clearest terms and in the most practical manner, everything I ever wanted to tell my father. How proud I was of him; how proud I was of being his son. Of the three children, I was always considered the one who was "just like your father" and I told him how that made me glow whenever I heard it, that I walked a little taller and held my head a little higher. I thanked him for his devotion to us kids, and for his devotion to Mom (recalling a quote I read somewhere that the best thing a father can do for his children is to love their mother). I thanked him for his lessons on life, his discipline and the opportunities he bestowed upon us; I thanked him for the time we spent together, whether sailing, flying, vacationing, or just hanging around the house. I thanked him for absolutely everything I could think of, and then I told him I loved him, that I loved him more than anything, and that he meant the world to me.

I cried as I wrote, and found the act of putting my feelings and emotions into words to be astonishingly therapeutic. When I landed in Singapore, I stamped the letter and dropped it in the mail. Everything about it seemed apropos: a letter on airline stationery, penned in flight on the very plane he flew, posted from a foreign country. About a week later, I called home to check in. My father, hardly loquacious or liberal with his emotions, let me know in his own way that he had received my letter.

When Dad passed away, he was at home surrounded by his wife of twenty-seven years and his three children. Not long afterwards, our family reconvened at the house to organize his belongings and prepare for life without him.

I entered his den to see what I could pack. There sat his small black duffle bag.

It was emotional just to see it, let alone open it. Pulling the top zipper revealed his personal items and the strong, sweet smell of his favorite tobacco, evoking a rush of nostalgia. I hesitated to touch anything and, after a few seconds, unzipped one of the side pockets instead. There, tucked neatly away, was my letter to him, which by all indications looked as if it had been unfolded, read and re-folded a number of times.

At that moment, I realized that my dad knew, right up until the day he died, exactly how I felt about him. Fourteen years later, this thought still comforts me and I suspect it always will—just because I took the time to write a letter.

~Christopher Bodell

68

One in Infinity

T hree years ago, while totally fatigued in summer school, I crashed my head against my desk. The impact caused my pink eraser to tumble to the floor, and the boy sitting next to me reached out to retrieve it. Now, three years later, he is my best friend. Together, we have tasted the sweet flavor of life. Together, we have realized that life is not sugar glazed—it is bittersweet, because without warning, life threw Raymond a curveball. Today, like tens of thousands of other people, he is battling leukemia.

During the end of eighth grade, I noticed that Raymond was slowly, but irrevocably changing. He was losing weight from his already thin frame. The boy who could once outrun me in any race now tired from quick walks. Moreover, even under the sweltering heat of the summer, he refused to slip out of his sweater. He claimed that he did not want the sun to tan his skin, but I later discovered that it was to hide the numerous bruises that covered his body. A year later, as we were about to finish ninth grade, he told me about the leukemia that was weakening his body.

"How long have you had it?" I asked him.

"Since I was six," he replied. His voice faltered as he attempted to meet my gaze. "It recurred last August, right before school began."

I flinched.

"There's definitely a cure, right? One that will make you healthy again?"

I grabbed his sleeve and tugged. "Why aren't you saying anything, Ray?" I already knew the answer. His hesitation was enough to confirm my fears.

"So, there's no cure?" I felt my heart plummet. If the world could have heard my heart pounding, the world would have heard the resounding beat of hopelessness.

"Helen, are you scared?" he asked. "You're scared, aren't you?"

"No." That was my monosyllabic response. Even though I only uttered one word, my own voice betrayed me. I wanted more than anything to sound brave, but I was scared. That day, I was so unforgivably scared.

By June of our tenth-grade year, Raymond's health had become so fragile that he needed to return to the hospital, maybe permanently. His visiting hours were short because the leukemia had sapped his strength so much that he could barely raise himself from his bed. His body was hardly responding to the chemotherapy and radiation sessions.

Raymond's only hope was a bone marrow transplant from a complete stranger, because his parents and his sister were not suitable donors. Although I never voiced my worries aloud, I often wondered: Would someone who never met Raymond before have enough compassion to save his life?

I cried that day, but what I remember most is that not a single tear had run down my best friend's face.

"My heart's still beating, isn't it?" Raymond said. "With every heartbeat, everyone slowly but definitely approaches death. The fact that my heart is still beating proves that I'm alive."

"Having a heartbeat isn't enough! You need to fight the leukemia, or else it'll never go away!" Those were the exact words I screamed at him.

He took a deep breath and murmured, "You don't understand life at all. It isn't a battle between happiness and sadness. Life isn't a fight for all or nothing! In fact, life was never a battle to begin with. Life is a story. People are afraid to die because they think they'll be forgotten, but it's not true! People exist even after death because of the loved ones who remember them. People are remembered because of the stories that make up their lives."

This was the profound reason he did not cry.

Was that what he thought life was? Just a story? I didn't understand what life meant back then. To me, life was merely being able to breathe. Raymond's definition frightened me even more than the leukemia. I was afraid that my memories would fade and that I would forget him. How long could stories last? Could they outlive memories?

Two months later, Raymond received a bone marrow transplant from an anonymous donor. An unnamed angel had given him another chance. With the complications of leukemia and the limits of medical science, Raymond only had a fifty percent chance of surviving after the transplant. Before I slept that night, I prayed for the very first time. I prayed for his heartbeat to stay strong.

But Raymond died of fever soon after the operation.

I was left with memories of our friendship—movies we watched together, days at the beach, random phone calls in the dead of night, and our idea to attend the same college. They all became a distant dream. I could explain my experiences with Raymond but they could never physically happen again.

At his funeral, I finally understood what Raymond had meant about life. It's made up of stories that are the very core of our existence. They are infinite and each one belongs to someone. These stories are told and retold, cherished, and treasured.

This is Raymond's story.

~Helen Luo, age 16

69

Chicken Soup
for the Soul

A Man's Best Friend

M iddle-aged men are not supposed to cry, but I did. The
phone call only confirmed what I already knew, that the
lumps I felt would be diagnosed as lymphoma. I hung up
the phone and immediately buried my head in my arms. I had not
cried like that since I was a little boy.

The cancer didn't strike me, or my partner, or any of our immediate relatives. It struck my friend, my best friend, a ten-year-old
Welsh Corgi named Mr. Fred.

I'd discovered the lumps beneath his front legs, all but hidden
beneath his thick coat of tawny fur, after he'd strolled into our bedroom and lay down beside the bed, waiting as he usually did for the
first tummy rub of the day.

It may seem presumptuous of me to talk about Mr. Fred's cancer
as if it were on a par with, say, a child's, a parent's, or a sibling's, but
just as there are many types of cancer so are there many types of
families. Not having any children, our dog is every bit a child to us,
his doting parents.

Our two-legged friends know we are taken with Mr. Fred, that
he travels with us when he can, and misses us when he can't. We miss
him, too, so we don't travel much.

They also know Mr. Fred is a very well cared-for dog. He visits
the vet regularly, gets all his shots, and takes his various medicines
and supplements according to a strict schedule. Corgis are prone to

disorders such as epilepsy, and Mr. Fred is no exception. He had one seizure when he was four, and he's been on Phenobarbital ever since. For the last six years his health has been excellent—until I found those lumps.

We took him to his regular vet right away, and within days she told us that he had lymphoma, but the prognosis was good because there were many treatment options, if we chose to pursue them. A specialist in canine oncology outlined a six-month program of oral and intravenous chemotherapy that would necessitate weekly drives across town.

The oncologist told us how much it would cost, but for my partner and I cost was not an issue that would prevent Mr. Fred from receiving treatment. If need be, we would have taken out another mortgage on the house. Thankfully, that wasn't needed, but the expense was a hardship we hadn't planned for.

For the most part, everyone understood. People who know us know we love our dog and would do just about anything to give him the happy and healthy life he deserves.

But one person didn't get it. She could not see the situation from our point of view, no matter how hard she tried, and we're not sure she even did. To her, Mr. Fred was a pet, plain and simple, and as such, as expendable as a stuffed toy, or perhaps a yard ornament.

"Why waste all that money? How could you?" Her voice was as upsetting as the original conversation with the vet. "There are so many more important ways to spend money! Why not give it to charity instead?"

Okay, charity is good, no question about that. But why would supporting Mr. Fred in his time of need preclude our usual charitable donations? We give generously to the causes of our choice. We would like to continue to do so, with Mr. Fred at our feet.

I wish we could have easily brushed off this person's insensitive comments, but it was harder than that. Not everyone has our view of animals, or knows how we feel about our dog, and that's okay. We wouldn't force anyone to share our way of thinking, and get along just fine with those who don't.

But this was different. She was family, and fairly close. She knew of our relationship with Mr. Fred. Her comments cut like a knife and hurt us both at a time when we needed to be as strong as we possibly could be, physically and emotionally.

I have to admit, I cried a little more, in secret. Dealing with cancer does that to you.

And, Mr. Fred could tell. Dogs behave in unique ways, especially when someone they know is hurting. And I was hurting. Maybe not as much as Mr. Fred, but enough that he knew. After that last phone call, he got up from his favorite corner where he'd been sleeping off a dose of Adriamycin and slowly walked across the room, his head bowed, eyes up, asking me what was wrong.

I couldn't answer, of course, because he's just a dog and they don't understand the things you want to tell them, about how you know he's scared when he goes to the oncologist every week, and you know the drugs make him feel bad, and you're sorry you're doing this to him but he'll feel so much better very soon.

You want to tell him these things and you try, but words fail, and you wish there was another way. Then his nose is against your knee and his warm little tongue is kissing your toes, and those big brown eyes are looking up at you from his furry face.

And you cry some more, but this time it's okay, because your arms are wrapped around him and your face is pressed against his muzzle and your hands instinctively scratch that one spot right behind his ear and he offers an appreciative little "woof" and wags his butt and you know that words don't matter because love is what it's all about.

And cancer does not weaken love one little bit.

~Daniel Molitor

70

Angels

I am a hospice nurse, working in a beautiful setting where every room has high ceilings, huge windows, and French doors that open to landscaped courtyards. I never imagined working in a place where beauty and death could share such close quarters.

My job allows me to experience events of the spirit.

One of these occurred with my patient, Imelda. She was in her thirties and dying from breast cancer, which had spread throughout her body. Everything had been tried to save or extend her life. She had a tube in her chest, and two drainage bags on her abdomen. She had been admitted for what is called "terminal care." This meant she would stay until her death. My job would be to keep her comfortable and educate her and her family as much as possible about the signs and symptoms of dying and death. The intention was to hopefully prepare her and her family, and thereby ease their anxiety through the transitions.

What I didn't know was how much Imelda would help me and everyone else involved in her care. I overheard other nurses speak of their conversations with her. She expressed gratitude at seeing another sunrise and being with her family. Light radiated from within her. Staff frequented her room. Every day, another priest or minister would come, loudly singing prayers in Latin and sometimes, Spanish. Although I couldn't understand them, the songs brought tears to my eyes.

I asked our housekeeper about the words.

"They're asking the angels to come and guide her."

During the few days I worked with Imelda, she changed. She wasn't so sure she was ready for death. She pushed friends and family away.

"Can we do anything else?" she asked repeatedly.

"Why do I have to have that catheter?"

"Don't help me, I can get up by myself."

She began to fight her lethargy and accused us of giving her too much pain medication. Her physician agreed to decrease her dosage as she wished, and even tried a different drug, allowing us to change amounts as Imelda requested.

Her weakness increased as her body declined. This went on for a few days. "You're still giving me too much medication," she complained.

I sat in the chair beside the bed and looked at her. "No, I'm not. Imelda, you are feeling sleepy because the cancer is affecting you everywhere. Your liver is not working well. Toxins are building in your blood. Your kidneys are also not working well. As these organs fail, you will get sleepier and more forgetful. Your body is beginning to decline." It was obvious by the look on her face that she did not want to hear this.

I continued. "Do you know what I'd be doing if I were you? I'd be spending time with everyone I loved while I could still talk."

She made no response. I left the room, unsure if her mind was clear enough to have understood all that I said.

Later that day, as I turned the corner toward Imelda's room, I ran into a crowd of at least fifty people, crammed in the hallway, coming to say goodbye. She'd heard me.

Our conversation replayed in my head as I drove home. I realized I hadn't seen my two closest friends in four years. They both lived in the same city, and it was an expensive flight. I always told myself I just couldn't afford to take the time off, let alone pay for the out-of-state flight.

Working in hospice, you come to realize the unexpectedness of death. You also spend many hours hearing the regrets of friends and family as they watch their loved one die. That evening, thanks to Imelda, I booked the flight for a long overdue visit with two wonderful girlfriends.

The priests came more often, singing prayers for Imelda. Her friends and family sat at the bedside, and patiently carried her from the bed to the bathroom, and back. At one point, we were unable to measure a pulse or a blood pressure, yet there she was, fully alert and talking with her family.

One morning I came to work, and the hall was vacant. Imelda had died just after midnight, with all her friends and family present.

It was during my lunch break that day that I noticed movement outside the door of our break room. I looked up and there she was, grinning. Her voice spoke into my mind. "Thank the nurses for me."

I responded silently. "You need to move on; please don't stay here."

Imelda laughed. "Don't worry, look who I brought!"

As she stepped aside, all I could see was an endless stream of angels. Shapes and faces blurred together, soft white and cloud-like. She giggled at the shocked look on my face.

"You need some help here." And then she was gone.

~Angie Edge, R.N., LMT

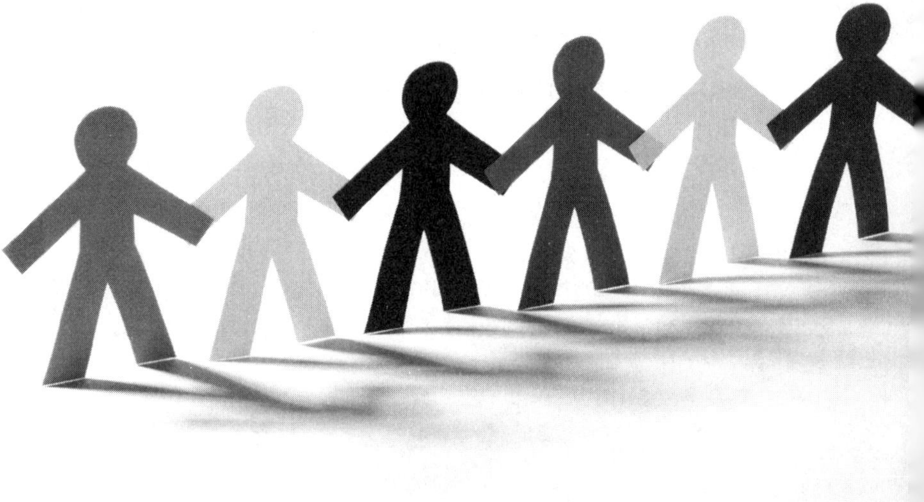

The Cancer Book

Fear and Hope

If children have the ability to ignore all odds,
then maybe we can all learn from them.
When you think about it, what other choice is there but to hope?
We have two options, medically and emotionally:
give up, or fight like hell.

~Lance Armstrong

71

Chicken Soup
for the Soul

Affirmations

"Is this where I get my underwear affirmed?" my friend Phyllis asks, as she walks into the bustle of conversation in my living room. We're having an evening of playfulness and healing, instigated by writing affirmations on our under- and outerwear.

I figure that positive words on clothing will help the inner healing process.

To begin, we sit in a circle and share a story about a piece of clothing that is or has been important to us.

Karen describes the slinky, silky turquoise and green paisley jumpsuit she wore all over Boston years ago, an outfit that made her feel sexy and free.

Ginny, a former fashion model, describes the blue Vanity Fair nightgown that her beloved little Auntie gave to her.

Nikki still loves wearing her dad's old cowboy hats.

One by one, the stories unfold, each one healing through humor and positive energy.

I am healing from a diagnosis of breast cancer and have a vision of wearing camisoles filled with loving, healing words.

• • •

When first diagnosed, I asked, "How could this happen to me,

Miss-tofu-broccoli-vegetarian-exercise-every-day-meditation-prayer-person? How could I have cancer?"

But soon enough, I saw my illness as a spiritual as well as a medical journey. I began reaching out to friends, gathering advice and healing ideas. I vowed I would listen to everything.

"I know a wonderful medical intuitive," a friend told me. "You should call her."

I had never personally met a medical intuitive so I was curious. She asked me to send a photo and six pieces of hair from my hairbrush. A week later, she called and gave me a reading.

"Dear, darling," she said, "Don't let them cut you. I can help you heal in twenty-one days. Give me twenty-one days."

"Does this mean the lump in my breast will be gone?" I asked her.

"Yes," she told me.

"And if it is not?"

"I will help you prepare for surgery," she said.

I was intrigued. Part of me did not believe her and part of me liked the concreteness of the time constraints. My doctor had said I could have six weeks to experiment before having surgery. I scheduled my lumpectomy for a week after the twenty-one day period would end and began my healing journey.

Once I decided to go with the intuitive's regime, I felt a sense of calm. I had a plan. After three weeks, I would have a sonogram and see if my lump had diminished or vanished. If so, hallelujah! If not, I would have surgery.

I gave up sugar, yeast, all prepared foods, fried foods, and more. I embraced a routine of supplements and homeopathy. I took herbal baths and rubbed my body with a cloth, proclaiming that I loved myself. I wrote everything down in a journal and tried to release old hurts and fears. I prayed and meditated, using imagery to see the cancer cells dissolving and flooding out of my body. I let myself be cradled by the kindness and compassionate caring of my friends and family.

On the twenty-third day, my husband, Ron, and I got on a plane to go meet with the intuitive. My hands were sweating when we stepped into the modern office building that housed her office. When we met, she hugged me and I felt her warmth and compassion. She ushered me into a small room, quickly scanned my body and told me she felt the cancer cells were fifty percent gone. Another six weeks of diet and nutrition, she thought, and they might be all gone.

I felt a little push of joy at the fifty percent reduction and a little stab of disappointment at the half that was still there. I left her office feeling buoyant, certain I would see positive changes on the sonogram.

The night before the sonogram, I prayed, "Please let me easily understand the results so I will know clearly what to do next."

The sonogram was taken under identical conditions as the original. My lump showed no shrinkage. Of course, the cancer cells could have diminished, but I could not ascertain that without another biopsy.

"The lump is the same," played over and over in my mind on the ride home. I had hoped for concrete proof that my healing efforts had worked. As I slumped against my seat, Ron gently reminded me of last night's prayer. I knew what to do next. It was time for surgery.

"Now it is time to surrender," a friend quietly advised me. "It is time to let go of the notion of control and go into the flow."

"Healing takes many different forms," another friend soothed.

I let the words sink in. The healing work had helped me feel strong, powerful, and purposeful in those confusing and scary early weeks. Following the intuitive's plan gave me time to research treatment options and shape my own healing ideas and hopes. During those six weeks, I felt flashes of nervousness and fear, but I never felt like a sick person. I felt vibrant and alive and full of promise.

In the days before surgery, my friends brought me food, prayer shawls, spiritual books, candles, soothing lotions, and fuzzy socks. I felt more open and heart-filled, allowing myself to truly feel and appreciate the outpouring of support, love, and empathy.

I remembered advice I had read years ago: When you pray, make sure you are willing to see the answer to that prayer in whatever form it takes.

I had prayed for healing. Though my lump had not disappeared in the way I had hoped, my prayers had been richly answered.

• • •

After sharing a potluck meal with my friends, we begin the affirmation process.

Ruth-Ann writes on a satchel in colorful, flowing script, "Leap and the net will appear."

Lori, who is also recovering from cancer, writes, "Limits are only in the mind" on a pair of gray flannel boxers.

Judith writes, "Giggle, Dance, Love" and draws a beautiful nipple on her pink T-shirt, in honor of her missing breast.

I have my friends write, "Healing, Dance, Sexy, You are loved" on my camisoles and feel the power of their words even before the paint has dried.

The entire evening is full of stories, laughter, healing energy, and hope.

Will these affirmations help me on my journey? I believe they will. Have my spirits been soothed and healed by the marvelous loving energy of my friends? Yes they have.

~Deborah Shouse

72

But I Feel Fine

I n August 2002, I was limping around with a sore and swollen toe. At night, I would tell my wife that the sheets were too heavy as they lay on my sore toe. Aside from the swelling that would come and go, I felt fine, so we weren't too concerned. I have my own paint and wallpaper business and I thought I'd been bitten by a spider while working at a dirty jobsite.

In September, my hand swelled so much my wedding ring had to be cut off in the emergency room. This swelling would come and go and I was tired a lot, but I thought I was just working too hard. My wife, Donna, thought maybe I had gout, a form of arthritis causing redness, stiffness, and painful swelling in the joints.

In January 2003, my jaw and neck became badly swollen so my dentist recommended that I see a doctor, but since I was never sick I didn't even have one. He made an appointment for me with a friend of his for the next day.

When the doctor ordered a battery of tests, we were a little concerned. When he told us he thought it was lymphoma and would be referring me to an oncologist, I was shocked. We never had thought my symptoms meant anything like that.

"But I feel fine," I said. "How could I have cancer?"

After that first diagnosis, things spun out of control. I had a biopsy, and began chemotherapy. I was hospitalized with pneumonia. I gave in to fear and depression. I could no longer work. I slept most of the time and was often sick. Yet, I knew I had to depend on God for the strength to continue each treatment, and He never let me down. After six sessions, my indolent (low-grade) lymphoma went into remission. I regained my strength and resumed my normal life.

In March 2006, I was itching all over and scratching so much I was creating sores, but other than that I felt fine. At my regular visit that month, the oncologist suspected a return of the lymphoma.

"But I feel fine," I said. Unfortunately, tests revealed the lymphoma had returned in a more aggressive form.

I think the most difficult aspect of the disease has been the questions, "Why this?" and "Why this again?"

I went through several months of discomfort before I turned the lymphoma to God. He had brought me through this once, but would He do it again?

I had to stop working, as I spent five days in the hospital every twenty days, leaving me weak and tired. Due to my compromised immune system, I could not go to church or anywhere large groups of people might gather. I was prohibited from doing one of the things I badly needed to keep my spiritual system healthy.

In order to decrease our debt and pay mounting medical bills we had to sell our rental properties, which we had counted on for our retirement. During one of my hospital stays, my wife ended up in a different hospital, fearing another heart attack.

I kept the story of Job in mind. He had many things taken away from him—health, wealth, family, and friends—but he still kept his faith in God.

I may never know the answer to "why this?" but I do know God has really used this illness to show me his love. Our friends and church family brought meals, ran errands, and spent time with me during endless days in the hospital. When I could not go to church, church was brought to me. An astounding number of people prayed for me and continue to do so. As my name and need are passed to many prayer chains, there is an army of saints I may never personally know interceding on my behalf. God has shown me that my spiritual family is larger than I could have imagined. The doctors and nurses have been amazed at my progress and I tell them, "Get used to it. I have a lot of people praying for me."

God has also taught me just how much I can trust Him. During the first bout we had no insurance. Some bills were decreased or cancelled, and the rest we were able to pay off when my wife returned to a full-time job with benefits. When the lymphoma returned, we were blessed to have insurance. It didn't pay for everything, but there were some treatments I would not have been able to have if the insurance had not covered some of the costs.

What we did not realize until the lymphoma returned was that there is no cure for this type of cancer. It is treatable and will go into periods of remission, but it is not curable.

When I am feeling down I remind myself that, "This too shall pass." A positive attitude does not mean no pain will find you. Sometimes there is pain. But a positive attitude and a belief in God will get you a long way down the road of recovery.

~Jim Paddock as told to Raquel Haggard

73

Chemo Hair

" "What are you doing?"

The last thing I expected to see was my little sister, lying sideways across the guest bed in our house, calmly running her fingers through her "chemo hair" and dropping hands full of beautiful silky blond hair into the wastebasket.

My gorgeous twenty-eight-year-old sister was losing her battle with brain cancer and accepting it with a grace and gratitude that blew me away.

Angel had always been very into her looks. I'm sure it stemmed from losing her hair at the age of three during her first battle with cancer. She beat that, but when her hair grew back, it was always very thin and she always fretted about it.

This past year, her shiny, silky blond hair had finally grown to her shoulders, but her pretty face had come to look battle-ravaged, bruised from constantly losing her balance (a side-effect of the brain tumor) and swollen from the steroids that she needed to help keep her brain from swelling. Her hair was no longer framing her face; it was simply falling out around her.

"What are you doing?" I asked again.

A little, half-smile lit her face.

"I'm thanking God."

My baby sis could see a blessing in every single situation.

I laughed at her upside-down pose, hanging off the bed, pulling out the rest of her hair and dropping it like it was nothing more than a disposable afterthought. I didn't know whether she was losing her marbles along with her hair, or was serious about thanking God as she lost her crowning glory.

"What are you thanking Him for, exactly?" I was puzzled, but knew there was a lesson here. I just had to wait for it.

"Because I have a chance to grow thick hair now!" She seemed surprised at my stupidity. "I've always hated my hair and now that it's falling out, I can grow new hair."

Most women I know, including myself, would be a lot more upset at being faced with losing their hair on top of everything else a cancer patient has to endure. For women, hair is a huge part of their identity.

I have always been known by my hair. I'm a redhead and have spent my whole life being called "red," "carrot top," and "that redhead." I don't think I'd know who I was without my hair.

But there was my sister, with an almost Zen-like acceptance of this new phase in her life, not only not hysterical, but feeling thankful!

She has taught me a lot.

The other day, Mom and I were running an errand and drove past the homeless shelter.

"Oh, they need potatoes," I said, pointing to the sign. "We should bring some."

Mom laughed. "You are so much like your sister." This was the highest praise I could ever hear and I glowed at her comment.

She continued. "One time when Angel was sick, we were driving here and the shelter had a sign out, saying they needed hamburger. Angel was quiet for a couple of blocks and then told me to go by her apartment."

Mom's voice caught at the memory. I clung to it like a life preserver, eager for more.

"When we reached the apartment, she insisted on getting out of the car herself," Mom said.

Shortly after Angel got sick again, she and her husband had

separated, an intensely painful thing for anyone, let alone someone fighting for her life. Her ex-husband kept the apartment and Angel moved in with me until she could no longer make it up the stairs; then she lived with Mom. Going to that apartment must have cost her dearly.

"So, he opened the door and looked at Angel with surprise. 'There should be some hamburger in the freezer,' your sister said defiantly. 'Is it still there?' He looked very confused, but told her it was, and Angel replied, 'Go get it.' Angel took the hamburger, and without a word, she left and I helped her back to the car."

"Then what?"

"'Go back to the shelter, Mom,' Angel said to me."

My sister, with her rapidly diminishing independence, often reverted to giving orders if she couldn't get the job done alone. It still makes me chuckle.

"By the time we arrived, Angel was wiped out and didn't have the strength left to take the hamburger in herself. I gave it to the ladies in charge and told them it was from my daughter. Angel slept the rest of the way home with no idea how amazing she was."

My sister never returned to the homeless shelter. The brain tumor took her life a couple of months later.

Unbelievably, she has been gone six years. In many ways, I feel like she was just with me yesterday. Things she did or said come back to me, often out of the blue. Her spirit of gratitude and generosity continues to bless me.

On days when I'm having a bad hair day, or feel cranky because of something superficial, I find myself remembering Angel thanking God on what could have been one of the lowest days of her life. Instead of going into a tailspin and feeling lost without her locks, she simply found the hope that comes with change, and from the deepest part of her heart, felt grateful for it.

Angel became a brilliant example of what God wants us to become during our time on earth. The biggest and best thing she taught me was this: Do what you can, when you can. Don't ignore the needs of others. Give a smile, comfort a heart, and feed someone who is hungry. And don't put it off, thinking you'll do it later. Do it now.

She never actually said those words. She didn't have to. She lived them. With what time she had, Angel used every bit of it, and then squeezed out a little more she didn't have, to manifest God's love for each of us through herself.

I think to myself that tomorrow I will get potatoes and gather up all the extra blankets and clothes we have at home and bring them to the shelter. I smile at the thought and then correct myself. I will go today.

~Susan Farr-Fahncke

Fear

had to get out of the house. My wife, Kathy, wasn't feeling well—again. Our son, Matthew, who is mentally retarded and autistic, was acting out—again, hitting, pulling Kathy's hair, throwing anything not secured, and banging his head violently. Tempers flared. Frustration was boiling over. I needed some distance. I could tell that Kathy needed it, too. After realizing that a relaxing Saturday at home was never going to happen—again, I snapped. I gathered up Matthew and his wheelchair and rushed out the door.

"Where are you going," asked Kathy.

"I don't know," I shot back brusquely.

"When are you coming back?"

"I don't know."

Cold.

I hurried Matthew out the door and into our minivan and sped away.

I drove with no real plan in mind. I didn't even know why I was driving. I only knew that something was bothering me. Something was making me incredibly angry. I needed to be alone to sort it out. But I knew that Kathy needed to be without Matthew for a while. He was safe to bring along for the ride. He can't speak, so I'd be free from interruptions and arguments.

Five hours later, I was still driving, still trying to figure out what was wrong.

Three years earlier, Kathy had been diagnosed with breast cancer, followed by a partial mastectomy and seven weeks of radiation. She had other ailments (diabetes, high blood pressure, and high cholesterol) which only compounded her problems. Subsequent tests showed no new signs of cancer, but for the rest of her life there would be invasive tests, careful watching, and anxious waiting.

Matthew was born almost twenty years ago and hasn't developed the same as our other sons. His disabilities and Kathy's cancer have profoundly affected our family and changed the course of our lives.

As I drove through town after town, I could barely begin to sort out my feelings as they collided with each other. Part of the time, I didn't even know if I would go back home. Of course, I had no reasonable idea what I'd do if I didn't. But at that point, thinking clearly was impossible.

A few hours later, Kathy called my cell phone. When I saw it was her I didn't answer. I just wasn't ready. She called again. And again. Each time, I was still too angry and confused to know what to say.

Sometime later, another call came and I thought I should take it.

"How are you doing?" she asked hesitantly.

"I don't know."

"Where are you?"

"Driving." I still wasn't ready for conversation or disclosure.

"When are you coming back?"

"I don't know."

"Are you coming back?"

"I don't know."

A long silence followed, both of us not knowing what to say, but not wanting to break the connection we had finally established again. We remained like that, on the phone, but not talking, for close to forty-five minutes. In that long silence, I turned the car toward home.

When we arrived, I brought Matthew into the house and got him settled. I still didn't know what to say to Kathy. I went straight to the walk-in closet in our bedroom and stood inside, not certain what to do next. Do I stay? Do I drive some more? I realized why I had gone to my closet. It was the only place in the entire world that was entirely mine to control.

Kathy came to the door and stood looking at me.

"Can you tell me what's wrong?"

Without thinking, the words shot out.

"I'm afraid."

"I know you are," she wisely replied.

It all began to become clear.

"I'm afraid that you'll get sick again. I'm tired of all the tests. I'm frustrated that there's always something wrong with your health. I'm afraid that I'm going to have to raise Matthew on my own and when I think about that, I don't know if I can do it. Sometimes, when I look ahead, it is just too much. So, I'm afraid."

There it was. Fear. I had finally recognized it. I had finally understood where the anger and frustration was coming from. And finally, we could talk about it, and we did.

As Kathy and I put Matthew to bed, the rest of the evening was spent opening our hearts, sharing our most painful fears and helping each other keep the darkness at bay.

~Michael D. Gingerich

75

Serious Foolishness

I was walking down the hospital corridor with a piece of toilet paper intentionally stuck to my clown shoe.

"Dr. Ginger Snaps!"

Ellen's voice was filled with urgency as she pulled me from the hallway into an alcove. She held me firm and looked at me through tear-glazed eyes.

"Tim is going down to have his leg amputated in about thirty minutes. He can't see me like this! Please can you be with him while I pull myself together?!"

My stomach churned. My chest tightened. I took my clown nose off to breathe a bit better.

"Please." She clutched my arm like she was falling off a cliff.

I nodded, but I felt paralyzed, scared, and trapped by her desperation. And, I definitely didn't feel funny.

I peered in through the doorway. Tim was sitting on his bed like Buddha. As he looked at me, I saw an old soul crammed into his seven-year-old body.

"Come in," he said. "I want to ask you something."

I cautiously tiptoed toward his bed, feeling consumed with dread. I stood next to him, unsmiling, waiting breathlessly for his next move. He slipped his little hand around my fingers.

"Do I have to go through with this?" he whispered.

We looked at each other, both of us hoping and groping for

an answer that would change everything. The silence continued. Usually, when it's clown time, a moment like that, stretched to its breaking point, is released with laughter. But not then, not with that beautiful boy.

I ached for something funny but it just wasn't there. Finally, I gave up.

"They think it's for the best, Tim."

He nodded with the kind of mature resignation a middle-aged man has when he receives the American flag in exchange for his twenty-year-old son who's been killed at war.

I couldn't bear it. I couldn't bear his courage.

Without even knowing what I was saying, I blurted out, "But we can do whatever you want for the next five minutes!"

Tim lifted his face and the aging man had become a boy again. His eyes twinkled with surprise and wonder. Our world was now alive with possibilities and we both chuckled like two little devils dancing at the gates of hell.

"Okay," he said with a puckish grin, "I want to jump on the bed!"

I looked at him for a second, confused, not getting it at first.

Of course, I thought, he's going to lose his leg! Of course he wants to jump on the bed!

"You got it buddy! Jump away!"

Tim started jumping on his bed, and after cheering him on for a bit, I got up on the other bed and started jumping, too.

We were breaking the rules and loving it! At one point, we were screaming and laughing so hard that his mom came in to see what was going on. She couldn't help herself. Our laughter was contagious.

We were all totally cognizant of what was about to happen. There was no denial. We just chose to surrender to joy instead of fear.

When they came with the gurney, Tim didn't resist. He calmly stopped jumping and laid himself down. I was so moved by his almost polite compliance, that I gave him my squirt gun to use at will on our way down to surgery.

Tim took full advantage. Sitting up on his gurney, he shot an unsuspecting intern in the hall as the elevator doors were closing. We all had a good laugh as the young doctor helplessly wiped the water off his shocked face.

Down in surgery holding, we made the anesthesiologist, his mom, his surgeon, and several nurses line up like ducks in a rotating shooting gallery. That was fun. That helped all of us get through an extraordinary moment in another ordinary day.

As Tim was being wheeled into surgery, he propped himself up on one elbow and yelled, "Hey, Dr. Ginger Snaps."

"Yes, Tim."

"You have toilet paper stuck to your shoe," he said, with a twinkle in his eye, knowing full well that I had put it there.

"How silly of me," I replied. "What would I do without you?"

Eventually, I would have to answer that question, because I've learned that moments like these never leave you. They are too powerful and too full to ever completely digest. Life is finite for all of us, and it is our task to find the joy in the journey.

This is my life. I am Karen McCarty, aka Dr. Ginger Snaps, professional goofball and hospital clown specialist—at your service.

~Karen McCarty

76

Can Lightning Strike Twice?

They say lightning doesn't strike twice. And yet, I find myself sitting in the same hospital where, nine years earlier, my husband and I sat, holding hands and pleading with God not to take our beloved daughter.

Sadly, that wish was not granted. Although we were both devastated, we were never bitter. We took the gifts of Jordan's life and death and let them mold us into better people, never taking anything for granted. We believed that our dues had been paid in the bad luck lottery. After all, is there anything worse than a parent burying a child?

So, how did we end up here again, sitting in the oncology clinic waiting room?

My husband, Rich, and I are the only two people here. Everything has happened so fast. I can't quite process it all. While we sit again, waiting, pleading with God, our six-year-old son, Zachary, is in one of the rooms with the pediatric oncologist, Dr. Halligan and his nurse, Peg, doing a bone marrow biopsy and a spinal tap to determine if our little boy has cancer.

My head is screaming. This cannot be possible. We already buried one child. We attend church regularly and we live a good life. God can't do this to us again, right?

I feel as if I might lose my mind. The pain in my heart is real. It seems as if it might stop beating. Just as it feels like the screaming in my head will come out of my mouth, Rich gently takes my hand and quietly talks to me.

"Mom, we'll do this, too. Whatever it is, we'll do it."

I can breathe now. Air has suddenly found its way back into my lungs.

"We can do this. We may not want to, but we will."

That one sentence would become my fallback over the next eight years.

They call Rich and me back into the room with Zach. Dr. Halligan is ninety-nine percent sure Zach has leukemia. They are sending his marrow out for a test, which will tells us in about four days exactly what kind it is. He tells us that we should hope for ALL. Although the chemo treatment can run up to three years, it has the highest cure rate, at almost ninety percent.

We move up to the oncology unit. As we are being brought to our room, I feel like laughing and saying this is a mistake. This just can't be right. We are all going to be so embarrassed later when the results come back saying he doesn't have cancer. Friends and family call over the next few days. I just keep telling them that Zach is sick. I won't say the "C" word. I refuse to admit it until I have proof. Even as they hang the first dose of chemo, I am still holding firm to my mantra. This can't be real!

But it is. The news comes. Zach has ALL.

How do you tell your six-year-old son he has cancer? I can't. Rich and I both chicken out. Dr. Halligan asks if we would like him to do it. We nod.

We follow him into Zach's room. I watch as this large man, with bushy eyebrows, and the kindest eyes I have ever seen, gets down on his knees besides Zach's bed. I listen to the conversation that will change our lives.

"Hey bud. Do you know why you are here?" Dr. Halligan asks.

"I'm sick?" Zach asks.

"Yeah, bud, you are. Do you know what you're sick with?"

"Cancer?" Zach asks back.

How does he know this? We haven't said anything in front of him. He can't know what oncology means. He's only six. Why didn't he tell us or ask us questions? Did we scare him into not being able to talk? We're going to have to do this differently from now on. He has to know he can trust us. We have to do this together. It can't be done alone. I slow my heart down and listen to the rest of the conversation.

"Yeah bud, you have cancer; you have leukemia," the doctor continued. "Can you die from leukemia?"

Oh my gosh! He did not just ask my six-year-old if he could die! I think I'm going to be sick. Last week, he was playing hockey. Now, he's talking about dying from cancer.

"Yes?" Zach replies.

"Yeah, you can, Zach," Dr. Halligan explained. "But I promise you I will do everything I can to make sure that doesn't happen. Okay?"

"Okay."

In that moment, Zach made a best friend. Through the coming years, Greg, as Zach would call Dr. Halligan, would be the driving force in what would keep Zach alive and willing to fight.

No parent should ever have to stand over their child's bed and wonder if they will still be there in the morning. We did that on more than one occasion. There was a brief eighteen minutes that Zach was in God's hands, and he handed him back to us.

• • •

Zach is now fourteen. He's in a wheelchair, on oxygen, and has a feeding tube. But he chooses to be a teenager who goes to school, has friends, and lives with laughter.

I choose not to be the mom of the boy with cancer. Instead, I am the mom of an amazingly strong young man, who continues to teach others to live life to the fullest.

That is our choice. What's yours?

~Tamara Kraus

77

The Butterfly Effect

t was a dream come true. I was about to see Paul McCartney performing at a benefit concert for Paul Newman's Hole in the Wall Gang camp—a summer sleep-away for children with cancer and other chronic, life-threatening illnesses. Among those joining the former Beatle that night was an array of superstars. But when McCartney came out to sing "Yesterday," backed by a string quartet, I was as if heaven had turned on every light.

Yet while the stars on stage were dazzling, the real superstars were the children from the camp who appeared both live and on film, fishing, playing, and even bantering with Paul Newman. One child even had the privilege of chatting with Paul McCartney onstage as the latter explained how "Yesterday" had come to him in a dream.

It was at that moment that I also started to dream.

As president of the Friedberg Jewish Community Center in New York, I have built and operated summer day camps for the past twenty-four years; in fact, my career began as a teen working as a counselor. But I'd never ventured into a medical setting. Yet, the more I watched and listened that night, the more intrigued I became. The questions kept running through my mind: Were there any day camps, as opposed to sleep-away camps, for these kids? Were any local? How many kids with some form of cancer lived in the area where I was running camps?

As amazing as sleep-away camps are, not every child is

comfortable in such a setting; nor is every parent able to make that leap. For children who are chronically ill, that hesitation can increase exponentially, often in proportion to the degree of illness. And even for those who are able to go, most sleep-away camps for children with cancer offer only one- to two-week programs.

What does a child with cancer do for the rest of the summer? What Paul Newman and others like him were giving to these children was a gift beyond measure. My question was, could my organization supplement such programs with a summer-long day camp where children with cancer would be able to come and go at their discretion? Keeping in mind the devastating effect that a chronically ill child can have on a family's finances, I also knew that if we were to offer such a camp, it would have to be free.

In a matter of weeks following this amazing concert, my staff and I were already gathering statistics and talking to hospitals. The initial response was overwhelmingly positive and we began gaining momentum at breathtaking speed. Soon, we had a general sense of what we would need to build such a camp, a place we were already calling Sunrise Day Camp.

We reached out to local supporters and to government officials to raise the necessary startup funds, while our Board of Directors voted unanimously to back the project. We assembled a team of advisors volunteer and professional, including parents, social workers, doctors, and child life specialists.

We visited Paul Newman's camp, along with others, to see firsthand what I'd seen on film, and more importantly, to learn.

We built an amazing team. Harvey Weisenberg, a long-time member of the New York State Assembly, agreed to be our honorary chair, while Bonnie Flatow, a veteran at Memorial Sloan-Kettering Cancer Center, became our hospital liaison. Michele Vernon, with a long career overseeing resident camps, came aboard as Camp Director and Adam Levy, Director of Pediatric Neuro-Oncology at Medical Center, volunteered to become our Medical Director.

Within months, four of the most significant hospitals in New York had signed on as affiliates, and a million dollars had been raised to build the camp. We rebuilt roads, put in misting tents and lifts for the pool, built playgrounds and sport courts, mini-golf courses and driving ranges, air-conditioned buildings and natural log cabins, and even constructed a universally-accessible tree house.

We opened with 106 children. A year later, four more hospitals signed on, along with 100 additional kids. This past summer, 266 children attended camp, with eleven area hospitals now part of the sunrise experience.

Sunrise Day Camp is a place where children with cancer, as well as their brothers and sisters, can enjoy being children, albeit for a day at a time. By the end of the first summer, we expanded into year-round services, and this year there are fifteen fun-filled programs planned throughout the school year. There are also family days, hospital visits for campers who have to be readmitted, and even programming within the hospital for children who are waiting for their chemotherapy.

And we're not stopping there. Sunrise in New York will continue to expand, and we are working with partners overseas to establish a sister camp in Israel.

We fill our camp with images of butterflies, as many of our children, whenever they've been hospitalized, refer to them as a metaphor for spreading their wings and regaining their freedom.

It also reminds us of "The Butterfly Effect," a scientific theory that allows for the possibility that a single small act, such as a butterfly fluttering its wings, can have an impact on events far greater than the initial act, and without the knowledge of the originator.

Without ever intending to, or knowing what they had done, Paul McCartney and Paul Newman set into motion a chain of events that led to the creation of a small miracle that has affected hundreds of children with cancer and their siblings.

The Beatles were right. All you need is love.

~Arnie Preminger

78

Chicken Soup for the Soul

A Woman's Choice

O ver my many years as an oncology nurse taking care of women with breast cancer, as well as my own personal diagnoses in 1992 and 1994, I have come to appreciate the importance of assessing a woman's feelings about her breasts before surgery. As part of this assessment, when first talking with a patient about her diagnosis and treatment plan, health care providers need to learn about each woman's relationship with her breasts.

How a woman reacts varies. One woman may say, "Take them both off. They don't mean anything to me." Another may say, "Will I have a scar on my breast after the lumpectomy? Will it be visible in the mirror when I look at myself?"

I often ask patients, "Tell me what you recall about the first time you were fitted for a training bra? Good experience or bad? How important are your breasts when you are intimate with your partner? If you were asked to rank your physical attributes, where do your breasts fall in that ranking?"

As a health care provider, this information can lend valuable insight into how well a woman is likely to cope with her upcoming surgery. Understanding a woman's feelings beforehand may help in her subsequent treatment. By anticipating reactions, you will be more successful at treating the whole person and not just the disease.

Facing my own diagnosis of breast cancer, I was no different than most patients.

I quickly discovered that having 44Ds on my chest affected part of my self-image. I faced mastectomy without the option for reconstruction—at age thirty-eight and again at forty. If it weren't for my husband teaching me that I needed to look at the surgery in a different way—as transformative surgery—I don't know how I would have managed things psychologically. He said the surgery would transform me from a victim into a breast cancer survivor.

After my surgery, I focused on being optimistic and was thankful that my life was being spared. I also learned that a woman's femininity is as much in her mind as it is in her silhouette. It is not based on breast ducts, lobules, and fat cells. However, having the privilege of being reconstructed ten years later reaffirmed for me that my psychological well being, though healthy, could be made better by restoring that which I lost to cancer a decade before.

A woman's relationship with her breasts influences her decision making about her breast cancer treatment, her emotional well being during and after treatment, and for that matter, perhaps even how much she fears getting this disease to begin with.

Culturally, as a society, we need to take a different approach when teaching our children and grandchildren more about self image. The values we impart should be tied to self-respect and the feminine strength that womanhood should represent.

A woman facing a diagnosis of breast cancer ought to inform her surgical oncologist and oncology nurse about her relationship with her breasts. Participate in the decision-making. Be sure the type of surgery you choose also addresses your psychological well-being. We each have the right to choose after careful thought, education, and planning. A year after a woman completes her treatment, I want to hear her say, "I'm happy with the treatment choices I made."

~Lillie D. Shockney, R.N.

79

Chicken Soup for the Soul

Fighting the God Fight

warm soft breeze played with the wooden chimes on Fiona's front porch. The flowers in her backyard were blossoming. Kids played in schoolyards, and dogs were joyfully chasing balls in the park. One beautiful spring day, Fiona was diagnosed with cancer and given a death sentence of a few months in which she would progressively wither away and expire into nothingness.

"You're my sister, and if you need a blood transfusion or bone marrow transplant, they can take mine!"

She smiled at me with a graciousness I had not seen in her before.

"I need more than a good fight, John." Tears sprang to her eyes and dropped onto her cheeks. "I need a God fight."

"What do you mean?"

"This is the fight of my life, for my life. I need God on my side."

I stared at her for the longest time. My rejection of a loving God had happened because of diseases like cancer—and all the pain and turmoil in the world—so I didn't know how to reply. I felt only anger and frustration that such a divine injustice could befall our own family. Why Fiona? Why not me, who defied God at every turn? She had a husband and kids. I had no one. Spare her. Take me.

But the cancer had laid its claim on Fiona and she had already made an important shift. She could do nothing about her diagnosis, but maybe she could do something about her prognosis. Who was I to question that?

"I'm here to help you," I said, intent on finding my own rock of Gibraltar amidst my tempestuous emotions. "May God be on your side."

Fiona began changing in many ways because of her illness, but most important, she learned to view herself differently. Lying in a hospital bed, she appeared more vulnerable than ever.

"How are you doing today?" I asked.

"Okay. Feeling quite a bit queasy, though."

"Did you eat lunch?"

"Didn't feel hungry." She hesitated. "I learned something new this morning."

"Yeah, what's that?" I took her hand in mine.

"Life is short."

I felt my heart breaking.

"And it's made shorter by a disease like cancer," she continued. "But now I know how to make it deeper and wider, if I get another chance."

I had managed to avoid crying until then, but the first tears of many rolled down my face that afternoon. Fiona had no regrets, no need to relive her life to make things better. All she wanted was more life. I silently raged again at a supposed God who could allow such pain to exist. If God is so all loving and all powerful, where was He now?

"How can anyone ever be ready to hear their doctor say they have a terminal disease?" she asked.

"I don't know."

"I was given a death sentence for doing nothing more than living my life to the fullest."

"And you're still here, Fiona, with God on your side, fighting." Even though I didn't believe in those words I knew she did.

Fiona believed in the power of faith—in herself. Where most people might sense a lack of control over their destiny, she found a new calling, to be stronger, braver, and more courageous than ever.

Where most people might only hear the sound of a terminal clock ticking deep in their subconscious, Fiona heard a more authentic voice saying, "It's not time to die yet. You have more living to do. This cancer is your reminder that you cannot take anything for granted."

And so, even when her body was betraying her, when it appeared that God had mysteriously vanished, Fiona chose to go deeper and wider and find Him again. I had lost God many times before and had stopped looking for Him but I fervently wished Fiona could find a miracle to save herself.

Would the cancer finally surrender to the treatment? Or, despite everyone's best efforts and prayers, would the treatment inevitably yield to the cancer?

Fiona hung on to a thread of hope that never snapped. Where she found the strength, I will never know. How she continued to believe, I will never understand.

One day, Fiona awoke and knew that the darkest hour of the darkest night was behind her. "I have two birthdays now," she announced. "October 20th is when I entered the world from my mother's womb. October 25th is the day I received my stem cell transplant, the day of my rebirth."

Fiona had been reborn in more than a religious sense. Her faith was confirming her new lease on life, which, in turn, was confirming her faith. As she said the day she returned home in full remission, "If life and love are not worthy of celebration, then what is?"

I had been reborn as well, but with new ambiguities. Could a person's newly considered faith in a God they didn't believe in actually be the lifeline to rescue someone from a terminal illness? Somewhere, on an island of rock-solid belief amidst an ocean of doubt, exists a world made in the image of the battles we wage inside ourselves.

By the blessings of her "God Fight," Fiona taught all of us how to live and love anew, deeper and wider.

~Joseph Civitella

80

The Fear of Hope

was standing under a tent on a windy fall afternoon with one hundred of my closest friends and relatives, singing, "To everything there is a season." It was the day of my younger daughter's Bat Mitzvah celebration. And, it was three days before I was to undergo surgery to remove a cancerous tumor in each of my breasts.

For me, the season was streaked with despair. The diagnosis of breast cancer had left me reeling. But it was also a season of hope and I didn't want to let cancer compromise that. The Jewish ceremony marks the start of a child's journey to adulthood. Like any parent, I dreamed of a wonderful future for my daughter.

Despite the round of awful cancer news — first a malignant tumor found in my right breast, then one in my left — my doctors had given me reason to hope. I was Stage II. The cancer had not spread to other organs. One surgeon said that after surgery, chemotherapy and radiation, I should have thirty more years.

"I want forty!" I told her. I was fifty-three years old at the time but I come from a family where eighty-year-olds are thought of as youngsters. But they're a bunch of pessimists, and I'm a pessimist at heart, with a dark side. When cancer burst into my life, part of me wanted to curl up into a little ball and feel sorry for myself.

But I knew that my two daughters, who were then ages twelve and fifteen, would take their cues from me. I wanted to show them that in a time of adversity, you have to face bad news with a strong sense of hope. I made a vow that I would not give into my negative impulses. I had a disease to fight. And a celebration to plan.

One friend said to me, "Of course, you're going to cancel the Bat Mitzvah."

But I had a purpose and a goal. Making the preparations for this milestone took my mind off the scary road ahead. I calmly told my doctors that any surgery would just have to wait until after Daniela's Bat Mitzvah. They agreed. My lumpectomies would take place six weeks after I was diagnosed, an acceptable interval in my case. But not a day longer, they warned.

On a beautiful Saturday in October, my daughter became a Bat Mitzvah—a daughter of the commandment. We chanted prayers, we sang, we danced, and we ate. Monday morning, I checked into the hospital for surgery.

As soon as I recovered from the operation, I began chemotherapy. Six sessions, scheduled from November through March, took a toll on my ability to hope. I was bald. I was exhausted. But I kept hope in my heart—hope that this awful ordeal would give me a future, free of cancer.

I'm a high school teacher, and I had decided I was going to continue working during the chemo months. Some thought I was nuts, but I wanted to maintain my normal life as much as possible. I even scheduled my six chemos for Friday afternoons so I would have the weekend to recover and be back in the classroom on Monday. When I felt up to it, I raked leaves, I went to the gym, and I went out with my husband, Marc. When I felt bad, I retreated to my bed and slept. Inevitably, I had to run to the doctor's office for pre-chemo blood tests and for shots to bring up my blood counts. Marching through my old routine at work and my new one as a cancer patient, I never really had time to think about hope or the lack thereof.

Then came my last chemo session in March. I was feeling particularly lousy. Marc finally convinced me to stay home from school for a day.

"Give yourself a little break!" he said.

What a mistake that was! I sat in the bedroom all alone and allowed myself to free associate, thinking the most morbid thoughts about my cancer. I wondered, what if all this hope and expectation of a good outcome was based on nothing? Didn't many other women go through treatment for breast cancer hoping that they would be survivors, and then, so unfairly, die of it in the end?

I realized later I was suffering from the fear of hope. Don't be too optimistic, and don't focus on all the characteristics of my cancer that made the doctors think they could successfully vanquish it. Because in the end you may be thrown the punch that none of us in the cancer world ever want to hear: So sorry, your cancer has come back.

Perhaps it's only natural that this fear of hope would bubble up as my treatments came to an end. I asked my oncologist if he would be scanning my body every six months to see if the cancer had returned. The sad truth, he said, is that catching a recurrence sooner rather than later does not have any impact on a patient's prognosis. What's more, scans would turn up all sorts of false alarms.

"If you are afraid to hope for a good outcome and it doesn't happen, then you won't have enjoyed the time you did have left," he explained. "And, if your cancer never returns, you won't have really enjoyed your life because of this worry and fear."

Easy for him to say. Hard for me to do.

I certainly don't think about cancer every day. But seven years later, I'm still fighting a war between hope and despair, my optimistic side versus my inner pessimist.

I wish I could be full of hope all the time. Life would be so easy. But then again, it never is. I think that's the message of the song we sang at my daughter's Bat Mitzvah, on the eve of my cancer surgery.

Adapted from the well-known Biblical verse, the lyrics speak of "a time to be born, a time to die, a time to mourn, a time to dance, a time to weep, a time to laugh."

There are times when I am afraid to hope. That's my nature, and a perfectly natural legacy for a cancer survivor.

So, I stay busy, I draw strength from everyone wonderful around me, and I tell my pessimistic self: There may be a time for despair, but there is always a time for hope.

~Marsha Dale

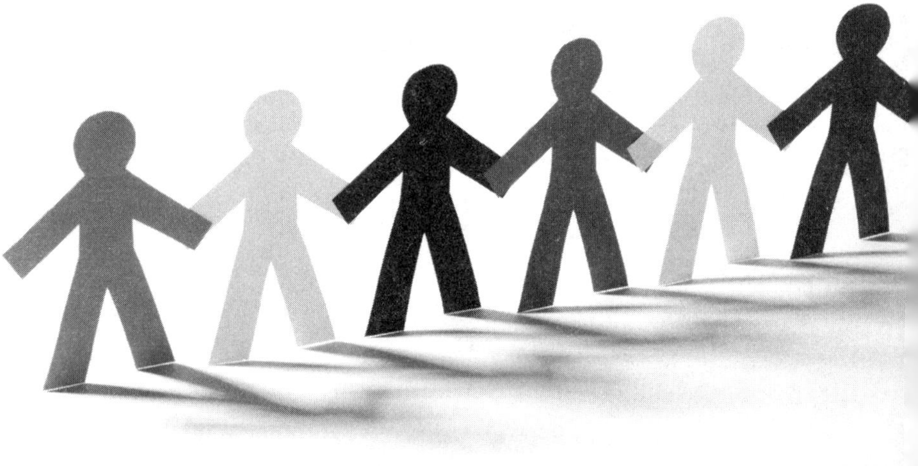

The Cancer Book

Letting Go

Let your joy scream across the pain.

~Ezbeth Wilder

81

Chicken Soup
for the Soul

How Nurses
Nurse Nurses

Two fashionably dressed young women meet by the water cooler while taking their morning break at the office.

"I guess you heard the news about Lindy?" The first young lady sighs, sipping daintily at her chilled spring water. "She found a lump in her breast."

"Oh my Gawd!" the second lady gasps, nearly choking on her water.

"Yeah, she went to the doctor and had a whaddayacallit, a mammogram, and they told her she has cancer."

"Cancer? But she's so cute and sassy! I can't believe it!"

Both women burst into tears and embrace each other. Neither of them says it out loud, but they're both thinking that they probably won't have lunch with Lindy because they won't know what to say or how to act. They return to their respective cubicles to contemplate the news.

Meanwhile, in a nearby hospital, two worn-out nurses stand at a counter, syringes in hand; one is drawing up 12.5 mg of phenergan and one is drawing up 10 cc of saline.

"I guess you heard the news about Carli?" the first nurse asks. "She found a lump in her breast. Had a mammogram and then a biopsy. It's cancer."

The second nurse flips the empty saline vial expertly into the trash with her left hand while her right hand reaches for an alcohol pad, a red top, a blue top, and a lavender top.

"How big was it? Has she had a CT yet? When will her path be back? I'll be back in a minute, I want to hear the rest."

Both nurses secure their materials and head off in opposite directions. Each of them is thinking of Carli. Both have a lot of questions.

That afternoon, Carli receives approximately fifty phone calls. She cries freely, laughs often, and tells her story over and over and over. She's telling us, her colleagues and friends, but also telling herself.

Carli schedules her port placement and lymph node biopsy. People she thought she hardly knew stop her with good wishes and promises of prayers and offers of donated vacation time and little gifts.

Grown men get misty-eyed and ask who is doing her surgery and then assure her, "Oh yeah, he's great, he's fine, he'll take good care of you." She is hugged well and often by a wide array of people. She volunteers to let all the girls palpate her mass so that they will know what one feels like. She says the men can too, but it will cost them in hard American currency, up front and no refunds. Carli laughs, the nurses all laugh, and then everybody cries a little until one of the men starts digging in his pocket for change. Then, everybody is laughing again.

Carli arrives for her procedure, calm and resolved. The hospital phone lines heat up as the morning progresses. Carli has her IV. Carli is okay. She is joking. She looks pale. Carli is in surgery. They are waiting for the preliminary pathology report. It seems as though the whole hospital is vibrating with anxiety and it seems funny to think that Carli is sleeping through it all.

The phone lines hum quietly, waiting. Finally, one call is followed by another, and two more, and four more, and then eight, until it is a wonder that the hospital lines are not overloaded and glowing red hot. Her nodes are clear, clear, clear, and was there ever such a beautiful word?

All over the hospital, prayers of thanksgiving are sent up, up and out. Carli has a rough road ahead of her, but she can do it and we will all help. And Carli, in turn, will help us to see how to be brave, how to have faith, how to love, and how to receive love.

And what about poor Lindy? I don't know.

For me and for Carli and for all the people we know, cancer is both less terrifying because we know a little about it and more terrifying for the very same reason. I have to trust that Lindy's friends will rally around her just as Carli's friends have. I have to hope that all the women and all the men who are diagnosed with some serious illness will learn what Carli learned in approximately one single hour—that they are loved, that they have friends who will help in all the ways that friends can, and that life is very, very beautiful.

~Elizabeth Bussey-Sowdal, R.N.

82

Chicken Soup for the Soul

Relay for Life

The running track is silent, with just the sound of moving feet. Each breath, each whimper or cry, strikes a cord within me as I make my way around, with my best friend at my side. I realize I am putting my weight on him but he simply readjusts his arm to better support mine. I hold on tight, not wanting to let the first tear fall. Once a tear falls, the floodgates open.

The luminaria ceremony is something to behold. The dark, cool sky is lit up by the bags lining the track, each one holding candles. I can hear the soft hum as they rustle in the wind. Every bag has the name of a hero to go with it, whether they are currently engaged in the fight against cancer or if they have passed on. I wish I could meet them, the people who were so loved. Cancer has cheated me of the chance.

I yearn for this day every year, ever since my mother passed away seven years ago. I treasure this moment, to be among the masses, all celebrating and mourning and grieving as one. I don't like keeping the sadness and the loss inside. If I do, it will creep up on me and find me. I need a friend to remind me of the warmth with a word, a smile, or a shoulder to lean on.

As I scan the names of the glowing bags, I fall upon a familiar one I made earlier in the night. It has my favorite picture of my mom and me from the scrapbook she made me as a gift before she died.

An *a cappella* group is humming some song about remembering.

All along, I can feel the warmth of my mom's touch. I would give the world for her to hold me again, because even at the age of twenty-one, I still yearn for that feeling. I know that comfort would allow me to release the anger and pain I'm still holding. I am angry that she left me. I am angry that my dad did not save her. I am angry that no one stepped up in her absence. I hold on to the thought that with her comfort I can let that anger go.

If only she could see the man I have become today, I think she would be proud of me. I have always vowed to carry on in her generous ways so her spirit would live on forever. I don't think I believe in spirits but I do believe in the love I feel inside from her.

It's empowering to walk among so many, to not feel alone in this struggle. I know I could turn anywhere and there will be someone ready to support me. The American Cancer Society's Relay For Life has embodied the celebration of life, remembering those lost, and fighting back year-round against this horrible disease. I am honored to be a part of this movement.

If you have ever cared for someone with cancer, you are a caregiver. It probably hasn't been easy for you, especially if you have been left behind to live on in this world. We survivors of a different sort are here for you—to listen, to cry, and to love. You are never truly alone. I hope you come out from the dark and walk the glowing track with me past the spirits that watch us, proudly.

~Daniel Wald

83

Chicken Soup for the Soul

A Good Goodbye

By the time I turned seventeen, I had already come to terms with the fact that my mother would die young. She'd been diagnosed with breast cancer when I was ten, and in the years that followed, I watched her go through chemo, a mastectomy, hair loss, remission, more chemo, more hair loss, and a brain tumor. Accepting that she would die was never a challenge.

But waiting for it to happen was difficult because my mom was stubborn as hell. The morning of her mastectomy, she pulled my ten-year-old self aside and told me that people who think positive feel positive.

"If you want to get better, you'll get better," she said. "I want to get better, so I will."

She said it so matter-of-factly, the same way you tell someone that you ran out of quarters so you're going to the bank. I figured she just said it to make me feel better, but seven years later, as my mom was still cracking jokes about "using the cancer excuse" to get out of work, I realized she had meant it.

Unfortunately, the same determination that had kept my mom alive eventually prolonged her suffering at the end, and it saddened me to watch her hang on when I was ready for her to go. I'd been fortunate to have seven solid years with her after her diagnosis. I'd had plenty of time to squeeze every imaginable road trip, hug, fight, and shopping excursion out of our time together before she passed away.

I was ready. My mom, on the other hand, refused to give up. She continued asking me how school was going even though she couldn't stay awake long enough for me to finish telling her about French class. She insisted on taking care of herself even though she was fast becoming just a shadow of herself.

Eventually, her liver failed and the doctor told us she would soon slip into a coma. I didn't know exactly what a coma looked like, but I imagined it would happen like it does in movies, and honestly, I felt relieved. It was the beginning of the end—a peaceful end—and that brought me comfort. I figured we would just wake up one day and my mom just wouldn't, and that a few mornings later we would wake up and she would just be gone. As I soon learned firsthand, comas actually set on much more gradually than that and my mom apparently planned on fighting it every step of the way.

A week after her liver failed, she still hadn't died. She was alive, but only technically. She was awake for literally minutes a day. Conversations, if she even attempted them, were brief. Her breathing was labored and her skin was severely jaundiced and smelled stale, as if her body had already moved on and was just waiting for her mind to follow.

"I'm running to the store," my dad said the next day after I'd come home from school. He barely got out of the house anymore, but things had plateaued and I think he needed time to clear his head.

"She hasn't woken up today, but they say she can still hear you. You should talk to her."

I nodded and my dad left.

"Hi Mom," I said. As expected, I didn't get an answer.

"School was good today. We rehearsed my one-act." I'd written a play and the drama department was letting me direct it. She would've been proud if she could hear me.

"One of my friends is in it." It still wasn't registering.

I leaned back and sighed. This wasn't the conversation I wanted to have. This wasn't the conversation I needed to have. I needed to tell her to move on, that we would be okay. I had long since come to the conclusion that my mom was not letting go on her own. Something was holding her back. Something in my gut said she needed permission to die, and somehow I knew she needed it from me.

"Hey Mom?" I said, and I immediately started bawling. I knew what I had to do but didn't know if I could.

"Dad and I will be okay," I said. "It'll be hard, but we'll be okay."

I rubbed her shoulder and bawled some more because how the hell do you encourage someone to die?

"I love you," I ended up saying.

And what happened next will stay with me forever.

It sounds like something out of a stupid, cheesy movie. To this day, I worry that people will roll their eyes at me because I know I would roll my eyes at them. It's just too perfect.

After I said, "I love you," my mom, who had been completely unresponsive for an entire day, actually opened her eyes, turned her head, and inarticulately but definitely, absolutely, and undeniably said, "I love you." And then her eyes closed and she faded away.

My dad came home to find me sobbing and obviously I told him what had happened. We tried to wake her up but she remained unresponsive for the rest of the night. We said "I love you" again and we asked her questions, but she was gone. She had slipped back into nothingness.

And at three o'clock in the morning she died.

To this day, I take comfort in the fact that my last words to and from my mother actually were, "I love you." I take comfort in the knowledge that we still had some tiny bit of control. My mother's faith kept her alive. My compassion helped her let go.

Cancer is terrifying, but we are not powerless and it isn't all ugly. Some of the most tragic memories are also the most beautiful. I will cherish this one forever.

~Jess Knox

From the Other Side of the Looking Glass

I am an oncologist.

When the modern era of bone marrow transplantation (BMT) began in 1968, I was a junior at the Johns Hopkins University School of Medicine in Baltimore, Maryland. Dr. Louis Lasagna, the world-renowned clinical pharmacologist, had guided me there because, in his words, oncology was where the most exciting clinical pharmacology was happening. I dedicated the next eight years of my clinical and scientific training to becoming a member of the Hopkins BMT team. It worked!

But my decision to pursue oncology didn't come easily. I knew that becoming an oncologist meant that I was going to be elbowing death out of the way as best I could and for as long as possible for the rest of my life. And death was going to win the vast majority of the time. Was that the kind of career I wanted to devote my life to?

One chance meeting after freshman year influenced this monumental decision. While doing research in the laboratory of the oncology ward, I thought it would be good if I started to interview patients as practice for the training that would commence in my sophomore year.

The first patient I saw was an elegant, sophisticated woman, forty years old, who had Hodgkin's Disease, which in 1967 was incurable.

She knew she was terminally ill and was in much discomfort, and she spoke mostly in whispers. The interview ended soon after I got the surprise of my brief life of twenty-two years.

Beckoning me with her index finger to come closer, as if to tell me something in confidence, she uttered two words I will never forget.

"Kill me."

I really didn't know what to say, let alone what to do. I'm sure whatever I said was certainly amateurish and definitely insufficient for her needs. This was my first clinical encounter with a patient and my first experience with imminent death. I quickly came to realize not only the physical pain but also the emotional suffering and mental anguish that a diagnosis of cancer produces. What a shock!

From that moment on, I investigated the life and experiences of medical oncologists. I spoke at length with my laboratory research mentor, Dr. Lyle Sensenbrenner, a member of the Hopkins BMT team. I asked him a question, which today I consider somewhat impertinent, but his answer gave me the insight and inspiration to go on.

I asked him what percentage of all of the cancer patients he had treated were dead. I got an answer that was forthright, heartfelt, and amazingly prophetic. He told me that ninety-five percent were dead but he had helped, in some way, big or small, each and every one of them.

With his positive attitude in an atmosphere of such sadness and negative outcomes, I saw why Dr. Sensenbrenner was satisfied with his career and could be happy each night after a day of helping people. Wasn't that what physicians were supposed to do? Wasn't there gratification in that? I developed a new way to think about oncology. It wasn't as awful as I had imagined.

What convinced me was bone marrow transplantation. It was exciting, and "cure" was a word rarely heard back then in medical oncology. Technically, BMT was difficult and patients went through quite an ordeal. But, if a career in oncology presented the prospect of beating death, it would be hard to resist.

Since I joined the Hopkins faculty in 1976, I've taken care of many patients and performed or directed many bone marrow transplants. Many patients have been given the hope for cure but many died in the process too, mostly from recurrent cancer.

It was exciting, challenging, and heart wrenching, but ultimately satisfying. I was able to go home each night, no matter what hellish things had happened that day at the hospital, with the feeling that I had helped my patients in whatever way I could, great or little. And that felt good.

Recently, I discovered how great the feeling could be when I crossed paths with two former patients.

While commuting into Boston to attend a Red Sox game, someone tapped me on the shoulder while I was waiting for the train. She was with a young teenage girl I presumed to be her daughter. When I saw her close up, I recognized her immediately and remembered our first meeting in the mid 1990s in Tampa, Florida. At that time, she was a recently married teenager who had just given birth to a baby girl but was found to have recurrent Wilm's disease, a rare cancer for teenagers and usually fatal if not cured the first time around by surgery and oncology care. She was just beginning her adult life as a wife and mother, and her prospects were grim.

We performed a transplant and I followed her for a number of years, during which time things were sometimes touch and go. In the long run, she did well. After moving away from Florida, I lost contact with her. When we met in Boston, she told me about her life since we last saw each other. The teenager was her baby girl from our first visit. The woman, so inspired by her transplant, had trained to become a nurse and had worked on an oncology unit for a number of years, kind of like payback.

I had helped her to cheat death, live a normal life, develop a career, and raise her own child! My feeling of happiness was intense (even though the Red Sox game was rained out).

Just a short while ago, I heard from another former patient, whose acute leukemia was still in continuous remission. I remembered that during the transplant hospitalization her very young son had gotten mad at me for "taking his mother away." As we shared stories of our grown-up children, I was awed by the twenty years we had been in contact and how vastly our lives had changed during that time.

I had helped this person to cheat death, live a full life, raise her children, and preserve her family! It was incredibly gratifying.

I am retired now and have time to reflect. I am very satisfied with what I have done with my professional life and the contributions I have made to the field. I tried to help each and every patient I saw in whatever way I could. Dr. Sensenbrenner's simple but elegant answer to my pivotal question was prophetic. I saw more death than one would ever care to know or hear about. Death wasn't a specter looming in the background that threatened life; death was the reality of life that cancer patients faced all the time. I grieved for each of my patients who died, but the fact that somehow I made a difference in their lives, as the tales of these two ladies illustrate, made it possible for me to go on, day by day, trying to elbow death out of the way and makes it possible for me to be happy every night for the rest of my life.

I am proud to say I have been an oncologist!

~Gerald J. Elfenbein, MD, FACP

85

Chicken Soup
for the Soul

An Unknown Angel

E
ven today, I remember how angry I was at the woman who came to my door one evening some twenty-five years ago.

While home on leave from the mission field where my husband and I had spent nearly fifteen years as missionaries, a routine physical exam revealed that he had aggressive metastatic colon cancer, which had already spread to his liver. Surgery revealed even more metastases. Our immediate heartache quickly turned to high optimism.

Phone calls and visits and letters from many friends who knew us—and many who did not, but had heard of our plight—offered overwhelming encouragement. Almost everyone had a marvelous story to tell of family or friends who had the same or similar diagnosis and were living many years later to tell about it. Our hopes were high and our personal faith encouraged us beyond measure. No depression or dark thoughts in our family, we pledged. Nothing to think of but how our miracle would come.

Then, that woman came to see me. I assumed she attended the large church that provided a house for us during our leave. But unlike those who came bearing promise and hope, this lovely woman handed me a small gift of food and said just one thing to me before she left.

"I know you are hearing so many stories of success. But if you are ever ready to talk with someone who doesn't have a success story to tell, please call me."

I was taken aback, stunned, and even angry. How dare someone speak to me of defeat! Why should anyone mention anything less than success? We were going to beat this. Everyone said we would. Stories of healing and remission flooded my mind.

I do not recall how I responded to my visitor; I only know that I did not ask her name again, and I never called to hear her story. I already had ours firmly written in my head and it was a tale of absolute success.

But while I dismissed the messenger, her message hovered quietly in the back of my mind, especially during my husband's chemotherapy and surgeries. In those somewhat ethereal settings, I would recall the words of my unwelcome visitor.

"All cancer victims do not have success stories."

As my husband's condition worsened and reality slowly set in, I began to feel less angry toward the woman, until one day it all disappeared. I came to realize she was attempting to prepare me for the worst. She knew I needed to accept that not all cancer victims survived. For the first time, I started to imagine a different ending to our own story.

Nine months later, we said goodbye to a husband and a father and a friend. Our hope and faith faded as cancer claimed this good man. It was only after I went home from his hospital deathbed that I recalled the stranger who had offered me a different dose of reality. I never saw her again and no one seemed to know whom I was talking about. I searched the church directory to find her but I could only offer my thanks from a distance. I consider her one of God's angels, sent to prepare me for what would come.

While I did not tell my husband about her message, I somehow know that he knew. He spoke bravely to our three sons, one by one. His message to them: "I have tried very hard to show you how to live. Now I hope that I can show you how to die."

And he did. Bravely.

Our pastor, Dr. J. Hoffman Harris, wrote of my husband's death in the weekly newsletter. "On one occasion, John Wesley was asked the secret of Methodism. He responded by saying, 'Our people die well.'" Dr. Harris went on to say that my fifty-year-old husband of nearly twenty-seven years had embraced that secret because he too "died well."

Cancer came to our house. We prayed that it would go away. We did everything medically and humanly possible to find a happy ending. What we received was the gift of peace, the promise of an eternal future, and a model for both living and dying.

I had walked with my husband and the father of my children through a dark valley, looking for a brighter mountaintop. Although we never reached our destination, a stranger reminded me that not every journey ends as we wish and we must accept that a life in God's hands will always go His way.

~Elaine Herrin Onley

86

A Time to Remember

"Is there any sightseeing you would like to do while you're in Boston?" Randa asked. Randa was the meeting planner of the three-day conference where I spoke.

"We'll have about five hours," she continued, "before you need to be at the airport."

"I don't know if you would call it sightseeing, but I would really like to visit the Dana-Farber Cancer Institute."

"We can do that." Randa understood my request. She knew that this hospital, affiliated with Harvard Medical School, was where I had nearly died nineteen years before, during an experimental bone marrow transplant, a procedure that had saved my life from the aggressive onslaught of recurring breast cancer.

I had only gone back to Dana-Farber once, two years after the transplant. The experience, however, was so painful I was sure I'd never go back again. But now I decided to give it a try, hoping I could give some of those painful memories a proper burial.

On this visit, instead of crying my eyes out as I had before, I was filled with thankfulness and joy. It was a time for me to reflect and to remember how far God has brought me from that once weak and fragile patient who fought for her life, to a life filled with meaning and purpose.

Just entering the main entrance took me right back to that frightening day nineteen years ago when a nurse pushed my wheelchair out those doors to the taxi curb. After spending more than a month in isolation, I had been terrified to leave the protective hospital environment. Deathly thin and slumped in my wheelchair, I had a mask over my mouth and nose to guard against infection and a scarf on my head to cover my baldness. I can still recall as if it were yesterday the way people turned their heads and stared at me.

Seeing Dana-Farber Cancer Institute was helpful, but as soon as we discovered the bone marrow transplant patients had been moved to Brigham and Women's Hospital we headed next door to that facility.

As I entered one of their sectioned-off transplant units, I witnessed the once all too familiar sight of a nurse putting on the protective jacket, facemask, and gloves before entering a patient's room.

Another nurse noticed us and said hello with a questioning look. I prayed we wouldn't be asked to leave as I quickly explained, "I'm from Pennsylvania and nineteen years ago I had a bone marrow transplant at Dana-Farber Cancer Institute. I wanted to come back and maybe see a patient through the door window to remember what I had survived."

She smiled brightly, "Sure." Then she asked about my procedure with questions like, "What drugs did they use on you back then?"

When I mentioned the name of one of them, she shuddered and said, "Oh my, they don't even use that on humans anymore. It's too toxic."

"No wonder I still need lots of rest," I said, feeling like less of a wimp. That one comment alone made me instantly feel better.

As we continued to chat, I was surprised by how genuinely interested she was in my transplant and recovery. I really didn't expect any of the nurses there now to care, as none of them had actually been one of my nurses during those weeks at Dana-Farber.

The other nurse exited her patient's room. "I pointed you out to her," she said, "and I told her 'See that beautiful woman? She had a bone marrow transplant nineteen years ago.'"

I reached for a tissue as the tears welled up. "Thank you," I said.

I knew exactly what seeing a long-term survivor would have meant to me during that time of uncertainty.

The other nurse, the one that Randa and I had been talking to, said, "I just want you to know you have made my day."

I looked at her wondering what she meant.

"Actually, you made my week," she continued. "Many of the patients we work with are quite ill and it's encouraging to see someone as vibrant as you after all these years."

I suddenly felt stupid and self-centered. I hadn't come to encourage the nurses. I hadn't considered saying "thank you" to someone who had not cared for me as a patient. Until that moment, I hadn't even thought about how few of us ever return to the hospital years after our recovery.

But now I had been given the wonderful opportunity to look this nurse in the eye and say, "Thank you. You have no idea of the positive difference you make in the lives of people like me!" I realized it wasn't about her being "my nurse," although she honestly had made me feel better. I was thanking her for all of us who have ever been cared for by a professional caregiver.

As Randa and I left the building, I expressed my deep gratitude to her for being willing to bring me back.

"And here I thought this trip was all about me," I laughed. "Not only was it a chance to recall God's amazing gift of healing in my life, this visit was about giving hope to a cancer patient and bringing encouragement to the caregivers who help us survive cancer. I'm so glad I came back!"

~Georgia Shaffer

A Letter to My Sister

Dear Mary Jo,

I remember taking a drive on Cromwell Bridge Road after Dad passed away of colon cancer. Although it was mid-morning, the moon was clearly visible in the sky. When I got home, I wrote a little poem about it:

Moon in the morning sky
Hanging by the strings of God
Waiting to be seen and loved
By everyone who sees and loves

You're kind of like the moon, Jo. I've never lived a minute of my life without both of you in it. It's a strange feeling knowing that soon the moon will be gone for good and there's nothing I can do about it.

A few nights after I learned you had cancer, I was walking a deserted beach on North Carolina's barrier islands. Nights that clear come only once in a blue moon. Looking up, I could see the Milky Way, cutting a swath from horizon to horizon. I had an instant of vertigo, a dizzying feeling that I needed something to hold onto or I might tumble into that glowing spiral of a hundred billion stars.

I wonder where you'll tumble when the cancer takes you, Jo. Will you be somewhere out there among the stars, or still here, drifting in and out of the minds of those who love you?

I remember when we were kids, Mom used to say, "When something is lost and can't be found, it's probably on the moon." I always liked the way that made me feel, like the treasured things I lost weren't really gone, just waiting to be found again. I want to think that you'll never really leave either, that you'll be out there somewhere, waiting for me to find you. Maybe you'll be on the moon, just like Mom said.

The moon was out that night on the beach. What a sight for sore eyes, Jo. It was like a golden peach rising over the Atlantic, glowing like the wick inside a deeply hollowed candle. I don't remember her ever being that beautiful before. She must have changed in some way, or I changed.

Not that I'm religious, like you. It isn't for lack of trying, I just never found God in a church. I'd like the comfort of knowing where I'm going and who I'll be with in the hereafter. But I think the universe is too mysterious to know those things until I get there. If someone really had those answers that would be huge for me, like finding heaven on MapQuest or being able to book a room by the pearly gates through Expedia.

I'm not trying to make light of what you're going through, Jo. Truth is, I envy the strength your faith gives you.

Saint Paul's First Epistle to the Corinthians says that faith, hope, and charity are the three virtues every good Christian should have. Pretty good choices, but why did Paul pick them out of all the virtues available? Why not empathy, selflessness, and a sense of wonder? I do have faith in goodness and I usually hope for the best. But after getting the news about you, the notion of Christian charity is a little harder for me to swallow. If the creator really wants us to be charitable, shouldn't he practice what he preaches? Would a charitable god allow my sister and her beautiful daughter to be diagnosed with cancer within weeks of one another?

I don't know the answer, but lots of people must think they do. The self-help shelves of most bookstores have no shortage of titles on the subject. I've read a few of them, but why bad things are happening to good people isn't a question I'm inclined to ask.

It's hard to step away from the dying tree to see how it feeds the forest. But it does. I think if bad things never happened to good people, maybe good and bad would no longer have meaning. Maybe our lives would have no meaning either.

I have to live in the moments you're still with me, Jo. No anger or regret, only gratitude. I think you want that too, because that's the kind of sister I'm blessed with.

I had a hard time deciding how to close this letter. I know you're having pain and I wanted to choose the right words help you through it all. But they all sounded so contrived—and what I'm feeling for you is so real, nothing I wrote measured up. And then I realized that words aren't all you need. Notes on a dulcimer aren't spoken; they're struck. And if they're struck correctly, we understand what harmony is.

There's a mockingbird that perches outside my bedroom window most every night. He'd make a lousy rooster because he always starts to sing before the sun comes up. Funny thing is, I don't usually mind being woken up by moonlight. His song is really sweet, Jo. I wish you could hear it. That's the only way you'd understand, because a song like that isn't meant to be described, only heard. Hearing it brings me joy.

You have a song too, Jo. You've been singing it my whole life. Take it from me; it's sweeter than a mockingbird's.

Mike

~Mike Sackett

88

Chicken Soup for the Soul

Life Is Good

After eight years of medical training, one would think I would feel at home in a clinic. Yet, the first couple of weeks were a zoo—learning alphabet soups like CHOP, FOLFOX and RAD-001, spitting them out like a pro to my colleagues, explaining them in everyday English to the rest of the world, supervising a clinic at full capacity while simultaneously attending to patients with chemotherapy reactions—and, apologizing fifty times a day for being late and still being sincere at the end of a clinic day.

In the midst of that, I met CC, one of my first patients as an oncology fellow. CC had a history of breast cancer and lymphoma and had just finished her first-line treatment for recurrent metastatic lung cancer. Expecting to see someone who was pretty sick, I was surprised to meet a quiet, elderly woman who generally looked well in her pink "Life is good" T-shirt.

I learned that this retired nurse was feeling pretty well, despite the recent chemotherapy. With a glimpse of pride, she told me that she continued taking long walks with her husband every evening, without any problems. Although CC did not ask many questions, she came across as a very intelligent individual. I couldn't help but admire her quiet and confident demeanor in the face of not one, but three cancers.

I casually commented about CC's "Life is good" T-shirt.

"CC always wears that," my attending said. "She either has stock in the company or she truly believes it."

CC laughed with such pride that I knew she had to be a true believer.

A couple of weeks later, I had to break the bad news: the lung cancer was progressing. I was not completely comfortable telling someone I had met only once before that the best treatment we could offer had a less than ten percent chance of success, but the discussion went smoothly.

CC was pensive. I desperately searched for some comforting words but before I came up with anything, she looked up and asked, "When can I start?"

I responded with a sigh of relief, "As soon as you get the medication from the pharmacy."

I encouraged her to call me with any problems, and she did. She developed a rash and was distressed by it. She called repeatedly and asked for a dermatologist. I tried to reassure her that the rash was a known side effect and would run its course. I compared her rashes to the pictures in the medical literature and wondered when she would feel better.

CC continued wearing her "Life is good" T-shirt (and attitude) to the clinic. She was skeptical at times, but she trusted me and continued her treatment. To my relief, her rash resolved on schedule.

A couple of months later, CC's lung cancer remained stable but her anemia had persisted. We hoped that it was only due to the chemotherapy, yet it soon became clear that her lymphoma was back.

This time, breaking the bad news was a little easier, as I had gained more confidence working with oncology patients. Also, lymphoma is more treatable than lung cancer. CC went through four cycles of treatment without many side effects and her anemia resolved beautifully.

Just as we congratulated ourselves for the accomplishment, CC's lung cancer took a turn for the worse. We tried another treatment without much success and CC became more symptomatic. She started having more pain in her chest, which was explainable by her diseases. What puzzled us was that she developed a rare but severe abdominal pain that brought her into the hospital approximately once a month for seven months. She would be admitted during the night and given pain medicine. By morning, she felt better. We ruled out heart problems and intestinal issues. We speculated that the pain must come from her cancer pressing on some structures, but we had no data to support that. It was very frustrating. Yet, each time I saw CC, she would cheer me up and say, "Well, I don't like to have the pain, but at least it's gone now."

Despite her treatments, CC's lung cancer continued to progress and our options were running out. One day, during her sixth stay for the same unexplained abdominal pain, I went to see her. Her CT scan from the previous night was not pretty. CC wasn't eligible for clinical trials due to her recent treatment for lymphoma.

"I should talk to her about hospice," I thought.

I walked into CC's room, sat down by her side, and explained the situation.

She nodded her head without much emotion, and uttered, "I know."

I patted her on her back, promised to be there till the end and left her room. I sat down with her chart to write my daily notes. On the last page was a scribble from my attending, with a plan to try one more treatment, even though there was only a five percent chance of response.

"You just made the worst mistake of your life, you idiot," a voice in my head screamed at me. "You gave someone a death sentence but she may be fine!"

Eventually, I decided to go back and apologize to CC for my "mistake." In my mind, it would somehow change the outcome if it had just been my mistake.

I found her sobbing quietly. Before saying what I planned, I sat next to her and asked how she felt.

"I saw this coming," she said. "And I think I am ready. But it's still a shock."

I told her about the last treatment option and apologized. CC was neither angry with me nor happy about the news.

"I am a nurse and I know the chances aren't good. But I would like to try it."

She paused for a while and said, "I know you have tried, Dr. Lau."

I was simply shocked by all my conflicting emotions.

Despite her treatment, CC passed away before Thanksgiving.

I am so glad to have had CC as one of my first patients. She gave me the encouragement and confidence I needed to grow, both as a doctor and a person. And most important, she reminded me that life is short but "Life is good."

~Michelle W. Lau, MD

89

Chicken Soup for the Soul

The Rope That Binds

It was a gray November morning, when the fog gets so thick you can't see anything else.

I sat on the patient stool in the hospital shower, feeling like the fog outside had somehow gotten into my veins, overtaking my entire soul. I was so sick from chemotherapy and diarrhea. My hair was beginning to fall out. I felt old, alone, and very mortal. I was hoping a good shower and a hair wash would make me feel better.

As I turned on the shower, I noticed that the pressure was inadequate, to say the least. I guess the hospital didn't want to be responsible for drowning any of its patients, because I had never taken a shower with such little water pressure. But, as the water began to cover my body with warmth I did feel a spark of refreshment both in my body and in my spirit. However, when I started washing my hair, some of it began falling out and clinging to my body and I was unable to wash it off with the water running so slowly.

I sat there nude, humiliated, and weak.

I had already gone through a six-hour colon cancer operation and three chemotherapy treatments, and struggling there in the shower, I really, really panicked. I could not get the hair off my body or my hands. I almost pulled the panic cord but grabbed some towels instead. I wiped and wiped, trying to remove all the hair. I left a heap of towels on the floor as I crawled back into my hospital bed, feeling defeated. I felt very alone and disgusted. When the housekeeper came and had to pick up my mess, I felt so ashamed.

Cancer had caused me to depend upon other people in a way I had never dealt with before. I was always very self-sufficient, always the responsible and dependable one, always the one to do things for other people, and I never felt the need for anyone else's help, not for my basic needs, that is. But with colon cancer striking me for the second time in fifteen months, I had to depend on others for the bare necessities of my existence. I was terrified and depressed.

• • •

It has been almost four years since I sat on that little shower stool, naked and weak, but I still feel a loss of control over my life. I have handled my cancer by tying a great big knot in the rope of life, holding on for all I am worth, and waiting for the next shoe to fall.

"Is this any way to live life?" I question myself. The answer should be "no" but I'm sure I will never be the same as I was before cancer struck. I have returned to a normal lifestyle but I feel a seriousness about life which I never felt before. I try to tell other people that mortality is very serious and real but they tend to look at me with blank eyes, denying their own deaths. But I can't deny nor ignore my own mortality. I have looked it straight in the face. I understand that someday my lifeless body will be laying in the dark on some hard, cold table.

I have also realized a strong and positive lesson from my long and difficult fight with colon cancer. I have complete control over the legacy I will be leaving my family and I live each day in a manner which will bind me to them forever.

I want to share as many positive experiences with my family as possible. We laugh together—at a dinner theater, a theme park, a Saturday afternoon picnic, or just a night of pizza and TV. All of these activities take time and effort, and sometimes when I get home from a busy workday I am very tired, but all I have to do is look into their beautiful eyes and know that no matter how tired I might be, I will not let them down or lose any time I can share with them.

Cancer is a horrible, deadly disease and it has been the most painful and heartbreaking thing my family and I have ever had to go through. I never really want to forget the experience because I never want to take anyone for granted again. Life is too short for that. And that great big knot in the rope of life I have been holding on to is now the rope that binds me to the love of my family.

~LaVerne Otis

90

House Call

"It's so good of you to come again, Doctor," Ellen says with a tired smile. "He loves seeing you." It's just my second visit since I came two weeks ago.

"The hospice nurse just left. She said it would be soon." Ellen averts her face from mine before leading me into the small living room. "Let me just tell Jake you're here."

The pretense for these visits is medical. I always bring my prescription pad, but seldom are medications needed. The hospice nurses usually handle all of that. Instead, I come for the patient, for the family, and for myself. Sometimes, it is simply hard for me to let go.

I sit down next to an end table filled with family photos. I'm drawn to one in particular: Ellen and her husband, Jake, impossibly young, Jake in an army uniform and Ellen in her wedding dress, both smiling and beautiful, starting off life together.

It is interesting to see their home, to have a chance to glimpse a part of the life they live outside my sterile office cubicle with its otoscopes and blood pressure cuffs.

Ellen returns. "It was hard to wake him, but when I told him you were here he perked right up."

Jake is in a hospital bed squeezed into their bedroom. He is so thin that the covers swallow him up. He vaguely resembles the man who has come to my office for the past eight years for a medley of treatment regimens, each working a little less well than the one that preceded it. But he still has his trademark smile and manages a soft, "How ya doing, Doc?"

Unlike the last time, when he kept me engaged in conversation for half an hour, he can only manage a few words before he nods back to sleep. I sit and watch his labored breathing. The hospice nurse is right; it won't be long.

I say softly to no one, "Jake, I will miss you. The eight years went quickly for me, too." Looking at him in pajamas now too large for his emaciated frame, I have what seems an unexpected epiphany. In God's eyes, no one is unknown, no one is insignificant, and everyone's passing is important. It seems obvious that Jake's life has some magnificent, but perhaps inexplicable, purpose. He won't warrant a long obituary or a memorial service in a huge hall, but he touched many, including me. I sit next to him, convinced that his spirit will live on, although I could prove it to no one.

In a few minutes I can feel Ellen standing behind me, and I stand up to leave the room. She asks me to sit down for coffee and I gladly accept. She thanks me again for coming, and says it was so wonderful I could make the time. I think to myself that I really haven't done very much for either of them, but I'm glad I came. I ask about the wedding picture on the end table, and Ellen tells me about a Jake that existed long before I knew him.

"He was irresistible. I remember thinking, here is my dreamboat." She goes from a smile to tears in the space of a second as I sip my coffee quietly.

When it is time to leave, she thanks me again for coming. I tell her to call if there is anything she needs. In the driveway, relatives or friends are coming down the walk, carrying dishes of food.

In my car, I try to navigate the side streets to a recognizable intersection. Only then do I turn on the radio. More war, a housing crisis, global warming, refugees and hurricanes: the news is deadening, mind numbing, more than anyone can grasp.

Feeling undeservedly virtuous and impossibly blessed, I pull into my garage, walk into the kitchen and kiss my wife, thankful for blessings I in no way deserve. She asks how my day went. I ask her to sit with me on the deck before dinner so I can try to describe my house call.

"They are just two ordinary people, with a jumbled up marriage like we have, people in love and even more so now that she is losing him." My recounting seems frustratingly inaccurate to me, but I go on.

"There is never enough time; the days go so fast."

I'm aware that I am talking in maddening clichés.

"Our days blow away like blades of grass in the wind, scattered and hectic. If we could sometimes capture that rare second of recognition of how precious love is it would be a great gift. And then, if after we felt its power we could just hold on to just a sliver of its awareness, instead of having it all slip away unseen through our hearts and minds to be swallowed up by credit card statements and petty resentments and by ambulance sirens and by things we either can't or don't know how to say."

Looking at our lilac bush silhouetted by springtime moonlight, I think to myself that we all know that our days are like blades of grass. But knowing it and seeing it up close changes the perspective.

Before going inside, I offer prayers for Jake and Ellen, for my wife, our children, and my friends. And I also send up a prayer of thanksgiving for the privilege of being able to make house calls because if I can only hold this lamp unto my feet, this may be as close to a mission field as I might ever get.

~Glenn Bubley, MD

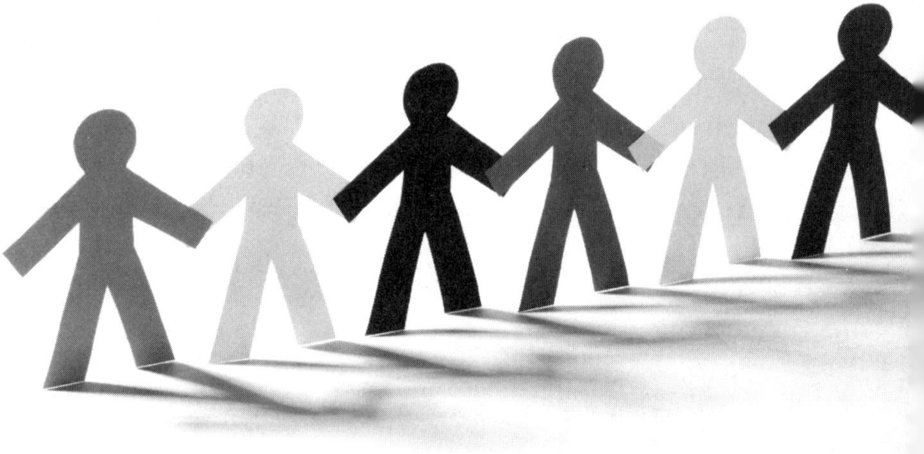

The Cancer Book

Into the Light

Love is the magician that pulls man out of his own hat.

~Ben Hecht

91

Chicken Soup
for the Soul

I Am a Cancer Patient

I am a cancer patient,
a mother, a wife, a daughter, and a friend.
I have a career and goals and a past filled with memories.
Sometimes, I wonder who will care for my children if I am gone,
Sometimes, I am certain I will live forever.

I am a cancer patient,
a survivor, an inspiration, and an advocate.
I have endured medical procedures and treatments
and felt exposed to total strangers in whose hands I lay my future.
I have moments of complete confusion and
        moments of total understanding,
nights of restless sleep and days of doubt and rage.

I am a cancer patient,
skilled at disguising any signs of illness with wigs and hats
        and make-up and smiles,
but do not be fooled—I am afraid.

I am a cancer patient.
viewed with pity and awe and a certain misunderstanding
by those who have not shared my journey.
I enjoy peaceful moments amidst the uncertainty

because I am acutely aware of life's preciousness.

I am a cancer patient,
a product of challenge.
I am thankful for the side effects that have helped me become
a better mother, a wife, a daughter, and a friend.
I am blessed to live life large.

~Amy Breitmann

92

Chicken Soup
or the Soul

Taking Nothing for Granted

My world came crashing down when I was eighteen years old and a freshman at the University of Richmond in Virginia. I had an emergency appendectomy and the doctors found a golf ball-sized tumor attached to my appendix. After the biopsy, the doctors determined it was Burkitt's non-Hodgkins lymphoma, a very rare but fast-growing cancer. They told me that the tumor could have killed me within a week. Ever since then, cancer has been a constant in my life. I am now a fourteen-year cancer survivor.

I was fortunate enough to take part in a clinical trial at the National Cancer Institute in Bethesda, MD. They are the best of the best. For two-and-a-half months, I basically lived in a hospital bed, receiving one of the most aggressive treatments available. In less than three months, my doctors gave me the same amount of chemo that most patients receive over nearly three years. I had twenty-four hour drips of Methotrexate, followed by Vincristine, among others. I had twenty-seven X-rays, seven CAT scans, six spinal taps (one that took two hours), bone marrow taken from my backside, a Hickman catheter inserted into my chest, platelet transfusions, and EKGs. I lost all of my hair and lost close to fifty pounds.

I had to be fed through a tube and took a wheelchair wherever I went. I started treatment so quickly I was unable to bank sperm and the doctors couldn't say whether I would ever get to be a father.

Nonetheless, I was so lucky to have a great support system. My parents, sisters, brother-in-law, and friends were absolutely amazing. I sometimes think a cancer diagnosis is harder on family than the person actually going through the treatment. It has to be tough having no control and watching your son, brother, and friend battling a deadly disease like cancer. I could have opened a Hallmark store with all of the cards and balloons that I received.

It was not all cheery all the time, though, because reality sets in just when you think you are cruising along. My third roommate had the same type of cancer as me and we bonded immediately. Unfortunately, there is a time when you are fighting cancer that you become neutropenic, i.e., you have no white blood cells to fight off infection. He started to get an infection around the same time the doctors noticed some white spots on my chest. White spots on an X-ray are not good. Turns out I had pneumonia. The doctors indicated they couldn't give me antibiotics since I had a zero white blood cell count, so they would have to wait and see. Meanwhile, my roommate passed away from his infection despite emergency surgery. I have never been more scared in my life, but I never, ever gave up hope.

I never really spoke about my cancer, since it was so easy to put it on the backburner and return to normal life as a college freshman. Unfortunately, it took my Aunt Joan being diagnosed with cancer, along with a good friend from high school, Ryan, who passed away, to wake me up to my own responsibility as a survivor.

In June 2002, I did a one-hundred-mile bike ride around Lake Tahoe for the Leukemia and Lymphoma Society's Team in Training. I did it in memory of Ryan and in honor of my aunt. This was my first exposure to the non-profit cancer research world. When I came down that final hill in Tahoe I had to pull over to the side of the road because I was overcome with emotion. I was crying like a little baby. They were both tears of joy and sorrow. I was happy that I had overcome so much and beat cancer, but sad that my aunt was going through treatment and that my friend had lost his fight.

That ride changed my life forever. It opened my eyes to so many things about survivorship. I also met my future wife that day while she was working at the Leukemia and Lymphoma Society. Our wedding was bittersweet because we knew that it marked the last hurrah for my aunt, who died a few months later.

Needless to say, I am very lucky to be here. I have become actively involved, not only with the Leukemia and Lymphoma Society, but with the Lance Armstrong Foundation. In May 2006 and the summer of 2008, I was fortunate to travel to Washington, D.C., with the Lance Armstrong Foundation. Our goal was to secure an increase in cancer research funding. I met with then-Senator Barack Obama's and Senator Dick Durbin's legislative assistants and discussed the ramifications of cutting funding. I also went to the inaugural LIVESTRONG Summit, attended the Presidential Forum on Cancer and have been actively involved as the co-founder of the Chicago LIVESTRONG Army.

Along the way, I have met some of the most amazing people. One of my inspirations happens to be a very close friend of mine, mountain climber Sean Swarner. I have been working with his non-profit, the CancerClimber Association for the last three years. Our mission is for patients and survivors to inspire one another by climbing their own "Everests" by giving adventure support grants to help them achieve things they never thought possible.

I am a firm believer that everything happens for a reason. Had I not been diagnosed with cancer, I would not be the man I am: brother, son, friend, husband, and most recently, father. My wife and I call Riley our miracle baby because I really wasn't sure if we would be able to have a baby. Riley brings a joy to my life that I never thought possible.

Life after cancer has been amazing. It's the best thing that ever happened to me. When I say this, I receive more than my fair share of odd looks, but I truly mean it. I have learned to take nothing for granted and as my friends, family, and wife will say, I rarely get stressed out. I don't really see a point in it. I guess cancer does that to you. I have so much to live for, so many things left undone, so many goals and dreams, that I would fight it until there was no more fight left in my body. Plus, I love surprises, good and bad, because that is what makes life so worth living.

Be well. LIVESTRONG. And Keep Climbing.

~Joe Schneider

My Learning Curve

t's the summer of 2000, one week since surgery. Part of my body's been cut away. The cat and I lay on the bed—she, with three legs (hit by a car), me with one breast. So simpatico I have to laugh.

I'm not a good patient. I don't want to rest—to do NOTHING. My identity is tied up with action. I am what I do. But I'm doing nothing. My world is so tiny right now, shrunken to fit in one chair and one bed. I haven't been outside in five days. I forget what's out there. My imagination is on the blink. All I know is fear and pain and so much love and concern from everyone around me that I'm absolutely floored.

• • •

Nearly a year later, on Mother's Day, I stand at the top of the steps outside the Philadelphia Museum of Art, my head covered in a bandana, hanging on to the arms of two strangers on either side of me. Scanning the crowd, I try to find my husband and children but I see my brother first, towering over everyone, tears streaming down his face. He and I had already lost one of our younger brothers and our father to cancer, and my breast cancer had reopened the raw wounds of those losses.

My thoughts are interrupted by the roar of 30,000 people in a sea of pink, cheering, as hundreds of breast cancer survivors descend the museum steps to begin the Race for the Cure.

Survivor. What does that mean? That's what I am now. What did I do that was so special? What allowed me to survive when so many others did not?

At age forty-seven, I'd had a normal mammogram. Three months later, I discovered a lump in my right breast while performing one of my sporadic self-exams. I'd always wondered how I would know if there is a lump, if I would recognize it. My question was unmistakably answered.

"How long have you been a survivor?" had become a routine question and I didn't know how to answer. Do I begin with the moment of discovery? Do I start counting from when I received my biopsy results on my cell phone, standing alone, listening to my surgeon?

"Bella, we found a little cancer."

"Just a little? Not a lot?"

Maybe my survivorship began when I slowly resurfaced through the fog of anesthesia after my mastectomy and saw the shadowy outlines of my family talking quietly and encircling me with love.

Did I begin to survive halfway through six months of chemotherapy when I'd wander around the house at three o'clock in the morning, feeling like a ghost and wondering if I had already passed on but didn't quite recognize it? Was it when I became filled with laughter watching an old Marx Brothers movie on the tube?

Throughout the year of surgeries and treatment, my favorite part of each day was after dinner when I put myself early to bed, exhausted after trying to have a normal day for my kids.

My daughter was eleven years old and my son was six. They'd snuggle in bed with me and we'd do homework, read, or watch TV. My husband would do the dishes and throw some laundry in the washer while periodically looking in on us. He was afraid to sleep next to me for fear of rolling over and hurting me. Sometimes, he would come in and hold me quietly while stretched out beside me.

One morning, maybe six months after my last chemo treatment, with my hair grown back and my schedule returning to normal, I sat and drank a cup of coffee while reading the morning paper. My husband had left for work and it was still too early to get the kids up for school.

I had been feeling restless and unsettled. All of my focus had been geared towards fighting cancer, beating cancer, cancer, cancer, cancer. Now, I was healthier and stronger as the effects of the chemicals slowly left my body. When the people I loved looked at me there was no longer a certain expression on their faces. I had gained back some weight. Things were getting back to normal. So why didn't I feel better? I seemed to notice obituaries for women who had died of breast cancer. What was the matter with me?

I read a story about a woman and her family who had allowed a writer and photographer into their home as she spent the final weeks of her life losing her battle with breast cancer. The photos were black and white, adding starkness to the images. In one photo, she lay curled up in bed, reading out loud with a small child on either side, the younger with his hand reaching up to stroke her wig, which later became a source of comfort for him after she was gone. In another picture, the family was on a beach. She looked so sad.

I lay my head down on the table, completely overwhelmed. I started to cry and I couldn't stop. I wailed in wave after wave of agony for that mother and her children and for the unfairness of this disease and for all of the wives and sisters and mothers and daughters who had suffered through it.

Finally, I lifted my head, and in a piercing moment of realization I was filled with the most unbearable awareness of what I had. How dare I not cherish it? How dare I feel sorry for myself? How dare I waste another moment of this life?

I woke up my children. I hugged them and kissed them. We had breakfast. We laughed, got dressed, and walked through town, crunching the dried autumn leaves on our way to school.

How utterly mundane it was. How utterly miraculous it was.

The first day I became a survivor.

~Bella Saltzer

94

Transcendence

Cindy and I were twenty-five years old when we married in 1965 and we had a wonderful thirty-two-and-a-half years together. When I asked her why she had chosen me from among her suitors, she said that I was the only one who had agreed to let her have twelve children. I assured her that I had misunderstood the question, or her intent. I had, however, "signed up for the duration." I let her down in the end, though. Time ran out on us after we had our tenth baby.

Knowing we would have twelve children caused me to leave public education and enter chiropractic college when Cindy was eight months pregnant with number nine. It was her support in raising our children that allowed us to live on a schoolteacher's salary as long as we did. It was her additional support that allowed me to work enough hours to support the family and attend school full time, eventually allowing us to build a chiropractic practice and share a wonderful life together.

When Cindy was diagnosed with terminal lung cancer (never having smoked a cigarette in her life) at the age of fifty-seven, our children ranged in age from fifteen to thirty-two. Four were married and we had twelve grandchildren.

To say the least, I was devastated. Cindy, on the other hand, was able to accept that she had done what she had come to do. She had "filled the measure of her creation." Sincere prayer brought me the peace I needed, with answers I could accept. The Spirit seemed to whisper to me, "No, you can't have 'that' miracle, but you will have others."

Three months into her four-month illness, our oldest daughter, who bore so much of the burden because she lived closest, asked me, "Dad, how are you doing it?"

I answered that I thought I was doing it about as well as I could.

She countered with, "Right words but wrong meaning. I can't believe how well you are handling this. The question is how are you able to?"

I told my daughter that I had come to know God of my own account at seventeen, and that I had never known Him to make a mistake. In fact, I had believed Him to be incapable of it. If Cindy stricken with cancer led me to believe that He had finally made one, I would have to change not only what I believed but also what and who I was. That was something I was not willing to do. It was also something her mother would not want me to do.

Cindy died a peaceful death, believing as I do, that our love would transcend death and that our family would remain intact.

I have experienced the miracle of a second wife, Ramona, with the kind of love Cindy wanted me to have again. My children have come to respect her and to love her. I have seen Ramona's three children increase my family to thirteen, a full "baker's dozen," which is one more than Cindy foresaw. I have seen the miracle of all thirteen children happily married with forty grandchildren and still counting. I have seen the miracle of God's love in all our lives.

Yes, there can be life and love after cancer and death.

~John G. Watson, DC

95

Blessed

My family ended up in a better place because of cancer. The same monstrous disease that slowly drained the life right out of someone we loved also served as a compass pointing us toward a better life, the kind my husband and I really wanted for ourselves and for our three children, after all.

When we learned that my mother-in-law had lung cancer, our entire family was shaken, but we were hopeful that it had been detected in time to be beaten. With the harshest of chemicals and radiation, doctors and specialists punished the cancer, but in the process, my mother-in-law took a significant beating.

My husband was visibly shaken by her appearance during a weekend visit. He struggled with living four hours away from her when she was so sick. And deep down, despite his strong faith and unshakable belief in miracles, he realized that his opportunities to demonstrate his love to his mother might not always be there.

Thankfully, the kids slept the entire ride back to our home in the city. We talked the entire time about making the move back to my husband's hometown, so we could be present, so we could make the most of what little time might be left.

For so many reasons, this kind of a move did not make sense. Bret had a good job in the city. As a freelance writer, the opportunities to network and grow my business were bountiful there too. We were just an hour away from my family. We loved our church. We loved the idea that our children had the opportunity to live and learn among people from cultures different than their own. We were ten minutes from the zoo, a science center, an art museum, and the mall.

Some people thought we were being foolish. But once we made the decision to move, things fell into place so smoothly that we felt certain it was meant to be. Our house sold within two weeks. Bret's employer agreed to let him do his job from home. Career doors stayed open for me.

We moved to a house just five minutes away from Bret's parents. The kids were able to ride their bikes with more freedom than they'd ever known. They made friends, and so did we. The kids saw their grandmother nearly every day. She'd swing by the house to take them for ice cream. She read books and had fancy tea parties with our three-year-old, Charlotte. Carol adored her grandchildren, so having them nearby was a dream come true for her.

While Carol was in remission, we were all able to fool ourselves that this was going to last forever. We'd heard the doctors tell us that Carol's kind of cancer had a nasty reputation for returning with the intent to kill. But all of us, including Carol, chose to compartmentalize that piece of information. Collectively, we ate dessert first and pushed the unsavory vegetables around on our plates, hoping no one would notice that we hadn't taken a bite.

All too soon, Carol started coughing again. And she couldn't take a good, deep breath. The cancer was back, and all of the possible antidotes had been exhausted the first time around. All she'd bought with those first blasts of chemotherapy and radiation had been a little time.

Our final months with Carol were an exhausting blur, especially for my husband and his four sisters. Many times, a call in the middle of the night meant that she'd fallen again, or that she needed to be taken to the hospital. All of Carol's children tried to grapple with what was really happening and how they were going to manage it.

My husband and two of his sisters were there when Carol took her last breath.

When we told the children the next morning that Grandma was

gone, they wept. My son Harry's seven-year-old body was wracked with long, hard sobs. As grief-stricken as they were to lose Carol, I think they were just as disturbed to see their daddy crying. At that moment, and for a few days after the funeral, I started to doubt the wisdom of our move. Maybe it would have been better to stay far away, to shield our children from the acute pain of losing someone they'd grown accustomed to seeing every day. Why had we put their little hearts on the firing line?

Once in awhile, I toyed with the notion of moving back to the city, back to our comfort zone. But in the short time we'd planted ourselves among the cornfields, something had happened. We'd established roots in this new place. All of us had made friends. We'd grown accustomed to some of the little niceties that come with living in a small town.

People wave and say hello, whether they know you or not. If your dog runs away, it's pretty likely that someone knows where he belongs and will bring him back. We know our children's friends and their parents, too. We don't want to go back to our former way of life.

All this time, we were sure that we were the ones doing Carol the favor. We were the ones doing the giving. We were the ones making the sacrifice. But three years after her death, we know that the opposite is true. Carol's struggle with cancer pushed us to think less of ourselves, and in the process we've been blessed over and over again.

~Anne Shaw Heinrich

96

Five Minutes

When you pass seventy years old, as I have, most every experience leads you to say, "Been there. Done that." But this past summer, I faced a new and different challenge. While my PSA tests for prostate problems were normal, as they had always been, my doctor decided to do a digital exam. She frowned.

"I think I felt something," she told me. "I'm sending you for a scan and a biopsy."

The technician at the hospital just said, "Hmmm."

After a few days of worrying, my doctor called and asked to see me.

"They took five biopsies and found one was positive."

"Positive? For what?" I asked a little dumbly.

"Prostate cancer," she said quietly.

Cancer is perhaps the scariest word in the English language. My mother died young from cancer after years of incredible pain. I didn't want to suffer the same way.

"Don't worry," my doctor told me. "If you have to have cancer, prostate cancer is the slowest growing. Chances are you'll die of something else before then."

I'm not certain whether she was trying to cheer me up or make herself feel a little better about having to tell me some bad news.

I was first sent to a urologist. I asked whether I would have to have the whole prostate removed. I had heard about problems like incontinence, loss of any sexual pleasures, and so on.

"We don't operate on men your age," he said rather formally.

An oncologist gave me all sorts of choices. It was a very small nodule, just at the beginning stage. I could wait a year or two.

"If you find termites in one room of your house," I said, "you're not going to wait until the whole house is infested."

The oncologist suggested radiation, five times a week for eight weeks. She waited for me to decide. I agreed. The five minutes it took to seal the deal were the most important five minutes in my life. Radiation was not like chemo. No hair loss. No upset stomach or nausea. It would surely work.

"I wish it were always so easy telling my patients about their cancer," the oncologist told me. In that moment, I realized that there are tens of thousands of people every year who undergo those terrifying five minutes of being told they have a life-threatening illness and deciding what to try and do about it.

But there are many men who just sit home. So, to all men over forty: Get tested. Don't always rely on a blood test, alone. And, if anyone is going to give you the finger, let it be your doc.

After eight weeks of radiation, the little nodule was gone and my prostate had returned to its original size. The PSA was normal.

Those five minutes had prolonged my life.

~Werner Haas

97

Chicken Soup for the Soul

A Humbling Experience

had always been the one who made a meal for someone in need, or sent a card of cheer, or called, just to see how they were doing. My parents set that example for me early in life. But in 2007, when I was diagnosed at age fifty-five with Stage IV follicular lymphoma (a non-Hodgkin blood cancer) without any symptoms, my world of doing for others hit a brick wall.

Suddenly, there were friends and family everywhere wanting to do for me. I was overwhelmed. All I wanted was this cancer out of my body forever. That's all. Food? Sorry, not hungry. Need a ride to the doctor? Nope! I can drive myself. (They won't take my license away just because I have cancer, will they?)

People stopping by the house saw me at my worst with no makeup, thinning hair (and then no hair!) and teary eyes. Emotionally and physically, I was at the lowest point in my life.

Soon enough, I learned that the shoe was on the other foot. I had to begin letting others do for me what, under normal circumstances, I would have been able to do for myself. I had to also allow others to see me at my most vulnerable, and I needed to learn how to do this with grace, without embarrassment or shame. The person I was prior to this diagnosis was gone and I was determined to have the new "me" be a more improved model. It was very hard, but it did get easier as the treatments continued to weaken me. I saw how helping me made it easier for my friends and family to accept a situation which was totally out of their control.

But even though I was growing more needy, my desire to continue giving to others only grew more intense. I didn't have the energy needed to make meals for the homeless as I had enjoyed before (heck, many days I couldn't even cook for my own family) so I had to come up with new ways to fill the void.

I began to knit baby blankets for our Bundles of Love ministry at church. This kept my mind from wandering to the dark places of fear that are so prevalent during such a health scare. And the concentration that was needed to knit the intricate patterns helped with the dreaded "chemo brain." My strength wasn't the greatest but I was able to crank out five soft and cuddly blankets and each stitch was full of love.

I also made beautiful ribbon and pearl crosses, and as strength permitted, I wrote thank-you cards and enclosed one in each. I've been told that these crosses have brought great inspiration to those who received them.

But the biggest thing I could do for others was to pray for them. There was much time spent resting on the futon during the day and, as I didn't want my feelings of F.E.A.R. (False Expectations Appearing Real) to overtake me, I chose to lift others up in prayer, which in turn, brought me great peace. I have felt the power of prayer from others and I know that it's the only reason why I have recovered so well from treatments.

I felt the need to repay all my friends and family for all their loving deeds, kind words, mountains of cards, and most importantly, their prayers. Before I went to sleep each night, I said my gratitudes for the day and vowed to myself that when I regained my health, I would make it my life goal to "pay it forward" in ways that I hadn't done before, like getting involved with new ministries and missions to reach a broader spectrum of people.

I have been humbled beyond belief during this journey. I have learned the graciousness of acceptance and how to allow people to love me for who I am.

Many good things have come from this horrible disease of cancer, many things that I wouldn't have learned or experienced if I hadn't been diagnosed.

Life will never be the same, and for me, that is better. I am not just a survivor. I am a thriver! Life, itself, feels fuller and more beautiful. Relationships are deeper, especially with my husband, and are more intense. Life is good because I have been humbled.

~Lori L. Smart

Love Can

believe love can help in curing cancer!

I am not a doctor and I do not know of studies that can prove this. But I know it is true. I have experienced it in my own life.

When our family discovered that my mother had cancer, we were silent. Usually, our house is filled with noise—old melodies played by Dad, soap operas Mom watched on TV (with her running comments), my sister, Nidhi, chattering on the phone, and continuous humming and giggling from me. On that day, there was silence.

Always the dreamer, I found refuge on the terrace. Gazing at the skies, I wondered aloud to God if we would ever be okay again. When I came downstairs, I saw Dad sitting with Mom, stroking her hair with such tenderness in his eyes I could feel every trace of anxiety leave her beautiful face. My sister was holding Mom's hand. We all looked at each other and knew that this was not Mom's fight alone. Her health would not just be the responsibility of the doctors; it would be ours, too.

Fear gave way to determination. Anxiety yielded to hope as we turned our attention to conquering cancer, every cell of it, with love.

One of the reasons cancer is so scary is because the treatment itself is painful. Chemotherapy makes one feel sick in every sense of the word. Since Mom's cancer was at an advanced stage, her medicines would be very strong and the doctors warned us that her health would deteriorate quite a bit. Hmm! Is that so? We looked at each other and shrugged our shoulders, almost in unison, as if to say, "Let's see."

We didn't allow any negativity to touch Mom.

An injection? We countered it with a "love you" and by holding hands.

Negative comments? We responded with a hug and an expression that said, "This person knows nothing."

Tears on our cheeks? We followed them with much laughter.

Trouble sleeping? We were up, through the night, chatting, playing cards, and listening to Dad's collection of beautiful old melodies.

Loss of hair from chemotherapy? We had an answer for that too! We called Mom the "Bald and the Beautiful!" and she would giggle like it was the world's funniest joke.

The result? Mom's red cell count, which should have fallen tremendously, stayed almost normal, through all six rounds of chemo. While most other people take about a week to recover from side effects she took only a day. The doctors were awestruck! One actually said, "Mrs. Bajaj, everything is absolutely fine; please leave so we can check someone who is actually ill!"

Before Mom became sick, she had always placed us before her, our health before hers. Not anymore. She began to invest time in herself. Mornings began with yoga and healthy food and her days ended with meditation. She started developing a love for her body, which I had never seen before, applying nice smelling cream on her arms and looking for pretty clothes to wear.

One day, out of the blue, she said. "I love dancing; teach me a dance."

Something very beautiful was happening inside my mother. Would this beautiful change have the power to defeat cancer? Her tests came back all clear. In fact, her reports showed that her health improved from what it had been before she had cancer.

Today, three years later, my mother's hair is softer than ever. She dresses prettily and goes to a group called Helping Hands to offer hope to other cancer patients. Just seeing her radiating with love, I am told, inspires patients.

Mom tells them, "Love yourself. Love those around you. And love life. Believe that you deserve to live and watch how cancer slinks away."

I believe her wholeheartedly.

Love works. It helped cure cancer.

~Megha Bajaj

9139

Thanksgiving is my family's holiday of holidays.

Each year, more than twenty of us come together to forget differences and enjoy a meal in the company of relatives. The next day, we are worn out.

One recent November, my immediate family drove to a local park where we sat and talked, just the four of us, catching up on each other's lives. My mom, dad, and sister were in the car in front of me. The day could not have been more brilliant. A cool autumn breeze was blowing and the sun was high in the sky. I enjoyed the drive with my windows down.

At a red light, I noticed the license plate on my parent's car. It was a special-order plate my dad had given to my mom as a Mother's Day gift. It read simply: 9139. For my family and me, that number meant everything.

When I was eighteen months old, I was diagnosed with neuro-blastoma, a malignant tumor wrapped around my aorta.

"The size of a grapefruit," the doctor said.

My mom balled her fist and placed it over my heart, her hand taking up the majority of my chest. It was a tumor that large.

The prognosis was grim—a ten percent chance of living, and with that came numerous side effects from the treatment: loss of hearing, skin damage, and a weakened immune system. Hope was something like the wind, blowing farther and farther away.

My parents were so young back then and made decisions I cannot even fathom today. One night was particularly bad. We were at a hospital in Chattanooga. I was two years old. My white blood count was deathly low. My temperature rose above 105 degrees. We made it to the airport, along with a traveling nurse. When we landed in Memphis, they hailed a taxi. My mom was holding me, shaking. My dad, trying to comfort her, was in a panic.

"We have a sick child here," he said to the driver. "Please get us to St. Jude Hospital."

"Please hurry," my mom added, cradling me.

They've told the story with such intensity that it's hard not to imagine the cab as it bumped along down the busy Memphis streets. It's hard not to see the street lights whizzing by in streaks across the windows. It's hard not to feel the muggy, warm air of Memphis as they nervously rode in the backseat.

"Your baby will not die, ma'am," the cab driver reassured her. "Not here. Not while I'm driving."

My dad tells the story more jovially now. "I saw the speedometer reach ninety twice: once on the way to the airport and once on the way to the hospital."

There are other stories, like the time my sister came to see me and asked, "Why are there so many wires in him?" Like the time my mother walked with me, lost, through some of the roughest parts of Memphis, knowing this was not the way she wanted to spend her last days with her son. Or the time I had to have a biopsy taken through my back. The three-inch needle had to be so precise a doctor said I could be paralyzed if I jerked too much. (How can a two-year-old not fidget?) "I'll hold him," my dad said. And he did, upside down in his arms. He says I wailed and screamed. "But I did not let you move an inch. Not one inch." He held me so tightly his arms ached for two days.

Now that I am safe and fine and twenty-five years old, the terror of my cancer has slipped away into our collective memories. At the park that day after Thanksgiving, my family enjoyed our time together. My mom is now a kindergarten teacher and she had many fun stories to tell about her kids. My dad still works as an engineer and my sister is happily living in Atlanta.

There is no more thought about my cancer, just reminders of it here and there. The most difficult parts have been buttoned up within the minds of my mother and father. They, not I, have carried its burdens.

We all hugged (yes, my family gives group hugs) and said goodbye. I traveled back to grad school in North Carolina, thinking about my parents' license plate.

Today, the ID numbers for St. Jude Hospital cancer patients are five digits long, allotted in numerical order as the patients are admitted. On my last visit to the hospital, I said to the woman behind the counter, "I am 9139."

"Four digits, eh? You must have been a young one."

And I was. So young, I don't even remember much of my actual time in the hospital. I only recall return visits for routine check-ups. Even those stopped when I turned eighteen.

The strange thing about cancer is that it is not a disease. It is, simply put, my own body's cells reproducing in an abnormal way. It's as much a part of me as my liver or my eyesight. The cells that keep my heart going are the same rogue cells that, years ago, divided incorrectly.

That license plate means a lot to my family, mostly my mom. It's the only thing that embodies our family's rocky beginnings, which inevitably made us stronger. For me, it confirms with pride that I am their son.

I am a cancer survivor. I owe my life and my happiness to their strength.

I am 9139.

~Travis Eisenbise

The Moment

Everybody has a moment when you know nothing is going to be the same ever again, when one part of your life ends and another begins. This is when you know that the changes, for better or worse, are going to be coming hard and fast. You're on a roller coaster and all you can do is hope that your safety belt stays fastened and that you'll come out in one piece. These moments are what make us who we are, and I know I wouldn't be quite me without mine.

Growing up as the oldest of three children in Dwight, Illinois, I had quite an uneventful childhood. My family was a huge part of my life. I had one or two close friends, and that's all I needed. I was healthy. If I had to describe myself, I would say carefree. I laughed a lot.

Then came the moment.

During Spring Break '07 I became plagued with horrible headaches. When we came home from vacation, I got terribly sick and was out of school for a few days. All was well for a few weeks until I got sick again. I couldn't focus and was seeing double. My eye doctor ran different tests and I really wasn't paying much attention because I just didn't want glasses. He explained that my optic nerve was swollen, which was causing my double vision. He told us that's normally caused by a tumor.

Stop.

Freeze.

Rewind.

Tumor?

As soon as the doctor left the room, I burst into tears. I didn't know what to do. A million things raced through my mind.

"Am I going to die? Do I have cancer? Can they fix it? Now what? O God, Kate, my best friend, is gonna freak out."

Eventually, I composed myself.

We were sent to get a CAT scan, which confirmed that I had a mass in my brain. We were shipped off to a hospital in Chicago. It was about one in the morning and I had doctors surrounding me as I sat on a hospital bed. For six days, they gave me standard neurological exams and a billion other tests. Finally, I went home and waited to hear more.

They thought my tumor was a Stage II and less aggressive, but recommended I go for a second opinion at a children's hospital which specializes in pediatric brain tumors. Those doctors considered it a Stage III tumor, meaning more aggressive.

We chose the more aggressive treatment, but I figured that was just as well. I wanted to get that sucker out of there. I really didn't like calling it "the tumor" or worse, "my tumor," so I gave it a name. Gary. I think he got it worse than me. Gary was beaten down with daily radiation treatments and chemotherapy for six straight weeks. Not to mention the steroids I was on to ease the swelling he had caused in the first place.

I rested for a few weeks before starting maintenance chemo. It was a little harder, with a larger dose and another drug added to the mix, but it wasn't too incapacitating.

One of the worst parts was going to the hospital for check-ups. Since I'm under eighteen, I'm cared for in pediatrics, with kids of all ages, shapes, and colors. It's heartbreaking to see a tiny little girl, maybe four years old, with thinning wisps of hair on her head, looking swollen from steroids. Most of those kids are too young to even understand what's wrong with them but they deal with the disease, anyway.

Since all of this began, I feel like a light has been turned on for me. I realize now that no one has forever, and that we need to spend our time wisely, because you never know when you're going to get a swift kick in the butt to remind you of your own mortality.

I have discovered the power of positive thinking. It makes you feel better and people around you feel better, too.

I believe I will continue to grow as I encounter new experiences on this roller coaster. My safety belt is fastened, and while I don't have my hands thrown up in the air with the thrill of the ride, I'm definitely alright.

Everybody has a moment, and a lifetime to make the most of it.

~Taylor Gettinger, age 17

I Am a Giant

I am small but big.
I am weak but strong.
Mom took me to the doctors,
Said I have cancer.
Didn't know what it meant,
All I heard was,
NO HAIR!

But I was determined to live,
To be who I am today.
A survivor is what I am.
I am a child, a friend, a daughter.
I am five years in remission!
I am a cancer survivor!

WOOHOO!!!!!

~Sarina Smith, age 12

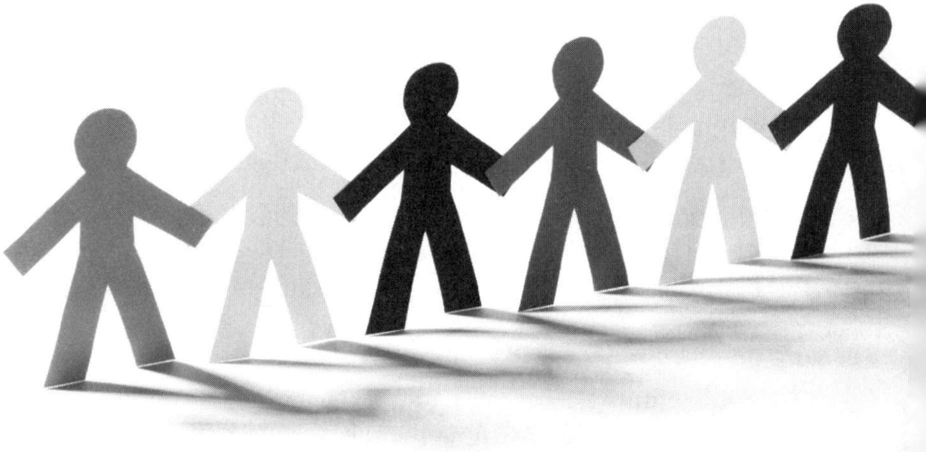

Chicken Soup for the Soul

The Cancer Book

Meet Our Contributors
About the Authors
Acknowledgments
Resources
About Chicken Soup
Share with Us

Chicken Soup
OF THE Soul

Meet Our Contributors

Megha Bajaj is the author of a book called *Thank You, Cancer*. Her entire life changed after her mother was diagnosed with breast cancer. Words like God, faith, and hope are no longer mere concepts, but have become significant realities.

Dave Balch founded The Patient/Partner Project after caring for his wife through five bouts with breast cancer. Visit www.ThePPP.org to access their resources for reducing stress and restoring hope for cancer patients and their families.

Emily Beaver is a fourteen-year-old girl in her first year of high school. She enjoys writing, acting, being with friends and family, and playing with her three dogs. She hopes to publish a novel someday. Please e-mail her at emilyb@cox.net.

Eleanor Bergholz has been a military spouse, an English professor and training director. She is happily retired with her husband, Richard, and lives in Venice, Florida; Falkenstein, Germany; and Clemmons, North Carolina. dick.bergholz@earthlink.net.

Rosalinde Block graduated from Sarah Lawrence College. She juggles multiple careers as a singer/songwriter/artist/illustrator/writer and teacher. She lives in New York City with her son, Joe. www.rosalindeblock.com and www.baby-wood.com.

Christopher Bodell is a finance professional living in New York City. He earned a Masters in International Accounting & Finance from the London School of Economics. Where his father's passing has left a void, his mother's love has more than filled it.

Amy Breitmann is Co-Founder of The Lydia Project, based in Augusta, GA, offering support and encouragement worldwide to women facing cancer. Amy is married to Troy and is the proud mother of Shelby and Mitchell. www.thelydiaproject.org.

Lori Brower, in partnership with the Empowered Wealth Foundation, does fundraising for cancer research and young adult survivor programs. She's an avid softball cheerleader for her daughters. She works with her husband, Lee, at Quadrant Living Experience, LLC.

Glen Bubley is an Oncologist, practicing at the same Harvard teaching hospital for thirty years, specializing in caring for men who are, for the most part, unsung heroes: prostate cancer patients.

Daniel Burns lives in Michigan, where he teaches fifth grade. He has a BA in Religion from Cornerstone University and degrees in English and Education from Grand Valley State University. Dan enjoys hiking, camping, and spending time with his family.

Elizabeth Bussey-Sowdal is the mother of four wonderful children, a practicing registered nurse, freelance writer, and speaker. She lives and works in Oklahoma City.

Al Cato received his Bachelor of Science from Florida State University in 1965. He is retired from IBM. Al enjoys being a grandfather of five, tennis, reading, and fishing, and is active in the melanoma support community. Please e-mail him at alcato@aol.com.

Amy Chmielewski is working on her Bachelor's Degree in Psychology from Cleveland State University. In the future, she hopes to attend graduate school in Clinical/Counseling Psychology. She enjoys spending time with family and friends. Please e-mail her at amyc441986@yahoo.com.

Joseph Civitella, MscD, is an ordained minister of spiritual metaphysics. He founded the School of LifeWork, has written *Shadows* *of Tomorrow*, and recorded the original CD, *Soulace*. He is currently working on his second novel, *Faith in Transcendence*.

Pete Collins is fifty and maintains an active lifestyle, despite a crippling injury in 1998. He's been active fighting cancer since his dad was diagnosed with multiple myeloma. He still bicycles more than 1,000 miles a year, kayaks, and dives. TheCrip58@yahoo.com.

Marsha Dale teaches high school ESL in Arlington, Virginia. She is the proud mother of Maya and Daniela. She missed her husband's company while he wrote the book, *Breast Cancer Husband*, but is glad he turned cancer lemons into lemonade.

Nisha Drummond, now a high school junior, lives with her parents, sister, and brother in New Jersey. She enjoys music, softball, and watching sports. She hopes to become a doctor and live in Boston. In May 2009, she will reach those five beautiful letters—C-U-R-E-D!

Christine Durbin is a Social Worker in West Lafayette, IN. Following her diagnosis of breast cancer, she worked to establish a chapter of Kids Konnected, a national group offering support services to kids who have a parent with cancer. cad5244@aol.com.

Travis Eisenbise received his BA from East Tennessee State University and an MA from the University of North Carolina at Greensboro in 2006. He now lives in Brooklyn, New York. He plans on pursuing a career in writing, whatever form that may take.

Gerald Elfenbein graduated from Harvard and did his clinical training at Johns Hopkins (MD, residency, and oncology fellowship) and his research training at the NIH. Retired from practice, he teaches, reviews manuscripts, and consults for industry and the law.

Liz Elliott is enjoying life with her amazing husband and two cats outside Seattle, WA. When she is not writing, she works with elders, gardens, and loves walks on the beach. Contact her via e-mail at laelliott@comcast.net.

Frank Emerson, a veteran, is a writer and award-winning singer-songwriter, living in Virginia with his wife, Frances, Director of Historical Resources for Wytheville, Virginia, and their Miniature Schnauzer, Simon. femerson@embarqmail.com.

Kelly Espy received her BS in biology from the State University of West Georgia. She worked in the science industry for fifteen years before making the transition to the nonprofit world. She currently lives in Minnesota with her husband and children.

Susan Farr-Fahncke is the founder of 2TheHeart.com, where you can find more of her writing and workshops. She is the founder of Angels2TheHeart, the author of *Angel's Legacy* and a co-author, editor, and contributor to more than fifty books. 2TheHeart.com.

Jamie Farris is an award-winning journalist and author. She is a full-time writer in the Pacific Northwest, currently working on her next anthology. Contact her at jamiefarris@hotmail.com.

Natalie Flechsig is a freshman in college, majoring in Political Economy of Industrial Societies. She plans to attend law school and become an attorney. Natalie loves to travel, learn languages, challenge people to Scrabble, and laugh. nflechsig@comcast.net.

Robert Gelnaw lives in NJ with his family, works in the financial industry in New York City, and spends most of his free time shuttling between his daughter's swim practices and his son's hockey and lacrosse games. Four years cancer free, he considers himself lucky.

Kathleen Gerard's writing has appeared in various literary journals and anthologies and has been featured on National Public Radio (NPR).

Taylor Gettinger is a junior in high school. She plays the flute in her school's marching band and enjoys family holidays. Taylor was diagnosed with a malignant brain tumor on May 1, 2007. She plans to attend college and pursue a career in teaching.

Michael Gingerich is an ordained United Methodist pastor and Director of Program Services for Cancer Recovery Foundation, www.cancerrecovery.org. He and his wife Kathy live in Hershey, PA. They are the parents of three sons.

Lindsey Goldhagen is a sophomore at University of Pennsylvania, studying to be a pediatric oncology nurse. Thanks to the amazing ladies of Phi Sigma Sigma and her friends and family, especially Wren, for keeping her alive. lindseyf@nursing.upenn.edu.

Werner Haas and his family escaped Germany just before Kristallnacht and grew up in Indiana. Werner published a novel, *The Wasps*, and worked with world-famous film director, Karoly Makk. He lives in West Hollywood, cancer-free.

Raquel Haggard is a freelance writer, living in Edmond, OK.

Joe Hayslett, Jr. was raised in Kentucky and earned degrees in Computer Information Systems, Logistics and Management. He's a Squadron Commander in the U.S. Air Force. Upon completing his military career, his goal is to publish books on leadership.

Anne Shaw Heinrich has been writing for more than twenty years. Her work has appeared in numerous publications. She lives in Dwight, Illinois, with her husband and three children. To read Heinrich's monthly column, *Small Talk*, visit www.thepaper1901.com.

Allyson Hellyer is a student at Indiana University. She enjoys writing poetry and hopes to have a career as a writer. Ally loves books, music, marching bands, and making people laugh. She owes all her inspiration to her wonderful family and friends.

Erika Hoffman's work has appeared in the *Chicken Soup for the Soul* series as well as in *A Cup of Comfort, Today's Caregiver,* and *Simply Blessed Christian Women's Magazine.* She and her husband have four children: Byron, Henry, Erik, and Heather. bhoffman@nc.rr.com.

Bonnie Jarvis-Lowe is a retired nurse. She is the mother of two grown children and a grandmother of one little girl, who all live in western Canada. She and her husband now live in their home province of Newfoundland and Labrador.

Pius Kamau was born and raised in Kenya and trained as a doctor in Spain and New York. Since 1980, he's practiced medicine in Denver, written a novel, and contributed pieces to *The Denver Post,* NPR and national media. He's just completed his memoir.

Barry Katz, inspired by his experiences caring for his late wife, Carole Singer, co-founded Lotsa Helping Hands, a free, volunteer coordination service, allowing a patient's community to assist during a medical crisis. barry@lotsahelpinghands.com.

Julia Singer Katz is originally from the Boston area and is currently an undergraduate at Temple University, studying social work. She plans on working with children in the foster care system. Julia enjoys sports, baking and her friends and family. Julia.Katz@temple.edu

Lauren Singer Katz grew up in Sudbury, MA, outside Boston. She is currently a senior at the Gallatin School of Individualized Study at New York University and lives in New York.

Andrew Kaufman is an Emmy-nominated writer/producer at KFMB-TV and KCAL-TV. He's completing his first novel and living in

San Diego with his five Labrador Retrievers, Jack Russell Terrier, and three horses. mail@andrewekaufman.com.

Jess Knox graduated from USC with a degree in Screenwriting and has written several horror stories about dating, which she's adapting into a screenplay. She interned with HBO, works for Omnipop Talent Group in L.A. and hopes to one day have an office.

Tamara Kraus lives in Schnecksville, Pennsylvania. She likes reading, traveling, and enjoying her family and friends. Tamara is helping Zach raise funds for St. Christopher's Hospital for Children. She is currently writing Zach's story. tamarakraus@aol.com.

Dr. Michelle Lau received her medical degree from Duke and completed her residency at Washington University. She's currently an Oncology Fellow at Harvard University. She enjoys traveling and plans to eventually settle in Phoenix, Arizona.

Bob Lenox is a full-blooded New Yorker who left town about twenty years ago to play music in Germany—and the rest is history. The idea of free medical care really appealed to a working musician and poet. Bob has three grown children.

Helen Luo attends high school in New York City. She aspires to major in medical science, with a goal of helping patients suffering from devastating diseases, such as cancer. Hobbies include violin, ice skating, drawing, listening to music, and her friends.

Debra Manford is a fifty-three-year-old grandmother, currently working with adults who have a developmental disability. Debra enjoys flower arranging, walking, reading, and photography. This was her first attempt at writing; the "phone call" was her inspiration.

Karen McCarty is one of the world's foremost experts on the burgeoning profession of hospital clowning and Associate Creative Director of the Big Apple Circus. Her memoir, *Serious Foolishness*, explores her battle with cancer and career as a professional idiot.

Mark McKinlay is Chief Scientific Officer of TetraLogic Pharmaceuticals, a biotech firm developing antagonists for treating cancer. He completed doctoral studies at Rensselaer Polytechnic Institute, and a postdoctoral research fellowship at Johns Hopkins University.

Ali Zidel Meyers was diagnosed with colon cancer at age thirty-three. Now thirty-five, she lives in California with her husband, Adam, and children Lev and Lyla. She is the Executive Director of Meyers Learning Center. ali@meyerslearningcenter.com.

Daniel Molitor lives with his partner, Ronnie, and their Welsh Corgi, Mr. Fred, in Pasadena, California. A graduate of the USC School of Journalism, his first novel, *Lair of the Jackal*, was published in 2006. The next is on the way. sonofgrecodan@yahoo.com.

Patience Moore is a Yale grad who teaches elementary school music. She's won awards for her family music project, Buckaroos Sleep Too! She's writing a memoir about her cancer experience. She lives in New Jersey and digs bicycling. www.patiencemoore.com.

Anetta Nowosielska is a writer, a pretty good cook, an adventurer extraordinaire, a loyal friend, and a carefree spirit. Working on her masters in creative non-fiction at NYU, she's a journalist who aspires to write the best darn book EVER. anowosielska@hotmail.com.

Elaine Herrin Onley served with her late husband as a missionary in the Caribbean. Following his death, Elaine worked in public relations. A published poet, author and artist, Elaine has three sons. She resides in Dothan, Alabama, with her husband, Ed Onley.

Joseph O'Rourke is a seventeen-year-old high school student in New York City who enjoys basketball, weight-lifting, math, and science. He plans to become a lawyer. You can e-mail Joe at segajojo@aol.com.

LaVerne Otis didn't begin writing until her mid-fifties. She's had stories published in *Country Magazine, Birds & Blooms Magazine*. Her hobbies include photography, reading, gardening, and bird watching. E-mail her at lotiswrites@msn.com.

Daniela Palik was born in Düsseldorf, Germany, and has lived in Berlin since 1982. She currently teaches dance and yoga and loves to travel.

Sharon Parkes received her nursing degree from SUNY and her Masters from the New School for Social Research. An Oncology Nurse at Beth Israel Deaconess Medical Center in Boston, she has a wonderful husband of thirty years and is blessed with four children.

Arnie Preminger is President & CEO of the Friedberg JCC in New York, and founder of Sunrise Day Camp. He holds a BA in Political Science, a Master's in Social Work, and received the Sofer (Scribe) Award for Excellence in Writing. apreminger@friedbergjcc.org.

Amanda Racette owns a marketing company in Buffalo, NY. She enjoys traveling, reading, writing, watching hockey, and fundraising for cancer research. Amanda and her husband, Nick, had their first child in late 2008. manda903@rocketmail.com.

Donna Reames Rich is an R.N., specializing in pediatric psychology. She lives in Florida with her husband, three daughters, dogs, cats, and the family hamster. She is working on a memoir and a children's book. donnachloe@yahoo.com.

Jonathan Rowe earned a PhD and MS in Biochemistry at the Albert Einstein College of Medicine and an MA and BS from SUNY. He is passionate about personalized medicine as well as his family and playing in rock bands. www.linkedin.com/in/jonathanrowephd.

Mike Sackett is a retired writing teacher and author of three novels and a children's book. His most worthwhile achievements are his daughter, Meghan, and face-painting children in Johns Hopkins' oncology wards. Contact Mike at sackettmike4@gmail.com.

Bella Weil Saltzer owns an interiorscape design business in New Jersey. She's been an actor and teacher of the craft for thirty years. In Maine each summer, she and her family love to kayak, stargaze, and make the perfect s'more. plantexpress5@comcast.net.

Nicholas Samaras won The Yale Series of Younger Poets Award for his first book of poetry, *Hands of the Saddlemaker*. Originally from Greece, he's a graduate of Columbia University and lives in New York. His writing focuses on the dignity of the human spirit.

Joe Schneider is an athlete, father, husband, son, brother, and fourteen-year cancer survivor. He has an amazing outlook on life and takes nothing for granted while living life to its fullest. Joe continues to show that if you put your mind to something, you can accomplish anything.

Hester Hill Schnipper is Chief of Oncology Social Work at Boston's BIDMC and a two-time breast cancer survivor. A nationally known speaker, her most recent book is *After Breast Cancer: A Commonsense Guide to Life after Treatment*.

Benjamin Schwartz received his Bachelor of Arts from the University of Pennsylvania in 1998 and is pursuing a Masters in Mathematics Leadership at Bank Street College. He teaches math in Manhattan, where he lives with his wife and children.

Za Zette Scott is a cancer survivor and mother of one son. She attended Jackson State University and works in the labor movement. Hobbies include reading, writing, and political activism. She lives in Upland, California. zazette1428@yahoo.com.

Georgia Shaffer is an author, licensed psychologist in Pennsylvania, certified life coach, and professional speaker known for her life-transforming messages to healthcare organizations. She speaks nationally to cancer survivors and general audiences. www.GeorgiaShaffer.com.

Lillie Shockney is an oncology nurse, breast cancer survivor, and Distinguished Service Assistant Professor of Breast Cancer, and Director of the Johns Hopkins Breast Center. She has published eight books and more than ninety articles and is a nationally-known speaker.

Deborah Shouse is a speaker and writer, appearing in *Reader's Digest* and *Newsweek*. She's donating proceeds from her book, *Love in the Land of Dementia: Finding Hope in the Caregiver's Journey* to Alzheimer's research. www.thecreativityconnection.com.

Cynthia Siegfried and her husband, Jim, have three daughters, seven grandchildren, and a very fat cat. They're co-founders of f.a.i.t.H., facing an illness through HIM, a support group for families fighting catastrophic illness (www.faithsupportgroup.com).

Cassie Silva is a playwright and children's theatre director from British Columbia. This summer marks her fourth year volunteering at Camp Goodtimes. She's currently adapting Kit Pearson's award-winning *Awake and Dreaming*. cassiesilva@ymail.com.

Marc Silver is an editor at *National Geographic* and the author of *Breast Cancer Husband: How to Help Your Wife (and Yourself) Through Treatment and Beyond*. His wife, Marsha, diagnosed in 2001, is today in good health.

Lori Smart is a retired Financial Aid Administrator from Northwestern Michigan College. She spent thirty years helping students improve their lives. Lori's passions are volunteering, working with stained glass, lapidary, RVing, gardening, and needlework. LLS102851@charter.net.

Becky Campbell Smith is an award-winning songwriter with twelve recordings to her credit. Becky has chronicled her family's story on www.caringbridge.org/nc/sarahsmith. She lives in Smithfield, NC, where her husband, Steve, is a pastor.

Sarina Smith is currently in the sixth grade. She loves to write and do art. She has been cancer free for five years, but is still dealing with the side effects of chemo.

Lauren Spiker created Melissa's Living Legacy Foundation, a non-profit for teens with cancer. She and her husband have six children and three grandchildren. They enjoy working in Melissa's garden. lspiker@teenslivingwithcancer.org.

Laura Strebel is a two-time cancer survivor who is self-employed. She's a cat mom and wife who enjoys everything about living. Her interests are varied but she mostly enjoys talking with other cancer survivors and helping them through the maze of treatments.

Sean Swarner is the only person in the world to have been diagnosed with both Hodgkin's disease and Haskin's sarcoma. A decade later, Sean became the first cancer survivor to climb Mount Everest. Sean hopes to give others the will to live and dream big.

B.J. Taylor is an award-winning author whose work has appeared in *Guideposts, Chicken Soup for the Soul* books, magazines, and newspapers. She has a wonderful husband, four children, and two adorable grandsons. www.clik.to/bjtaylor.

Elaine Truman is an Executive of the Professional Picture Framers

Association and Professional Scrapbook Retailers Association, head-quartered in Jackson, MI. She and husband Allen have three daughters, Erin, Elise, and Emmarie. trumaer@yahoo.com.

Emmarie Truman may be the niftiest high school student in the world. When she's not fighting brain tumors or pitching no-hitters, she can be found shoe shopping online or groaning over homework. Hobbies include photography, singing, and world peace.

Shereen Vinke survived a year of cancer treatment after graduating high school in 2001. She graduated from Calvin College with a degree in Elementary Education. After teaching several years, she became a full-time homemaker, enjoying reading, writing, and drawing.

Ken Wachsberger is an author, editor, publisher, and Eastern Michigan University writing instructor from Ann Arbor, Michigan. ken@azenphonypress.com.

Daniel Wald will receive his B.S. in biochemistry from Ithaca College in May 2009. He is an active volunteer for the American Cancer Society. Daniel likes to participate in outdoor activities. He is planning a career path in public health.

Pam Washek is the co-founder of Wayland Angels Inc., a non-profit providing help to neighbors in need during times of crisis. To learn about local communities in your area, or start your own, visit www.helping-angels.org.

John Watson became a schoolteacher at the age of twenty-nine, and ten years later he began his Chiropractic education. Following the death of his first wife, Cindy, he married Ramona Luker of Salt Lake City. Together, they share forty-one grandchildren.

Susie Leonard Weller has a degree in Pastoral Ministry and a certificate in Spiritual Direction from Gonzaga. She's a life coach and wrote

Why Don't You Understand? The Four Thinking Styles to Improve Family Communication. www.susieweller.com.

Charlotte Wheeler has been a nurse for thirty-seven years. She works as an Infection Preventionist in Amarillo, TX. She enjoys motivational speaking and gardening. She hopes to inspire others in their cancer recovery. char3223@amaonline.com.

Gretchen Whiting received her BA from U. of Washington in 1990 and her MBA from Cornell in 1998. She's a stay-at-home mom and volunteer in the Seattle area. Gretchen enjoys cooking, reading, walking, yoga, and spending time with family and friends.

Paul Winick, MD practiced pediatrics for forty-five years and is professor of pediatrics at the University of Miami School of Medicine. He and his wife, Dorothy, have two children and five grandchildren. Dr. Winick has published a memoir, *Finding Ruth.*

Rebecca Yauger lives in Texas with her husband and has two grown children. She was published in *Chicken Soup for the Soul: Celebrating Mothers and Daughters* and is on the board of American Christian Fiction Writers; writing her first novel. becky@rebeccavincent.net.

Matthew Zachary received his BA in music, computer science and sociology from Binghamton University in 1996. Cancer-free, married, and living in Brooklyn, he's proudly leading a revolution in advocacy for the young adult cancer community.

Jasan Zimmerman is a three-time cancer survivor, diagnosed with neuroblastoma in 1976 when he was six months old, thyroid cancer in 1991 when he was fifteen, with a recurrence of thyroid cancer in 1997 at age twenty-one. He writes because he needs to.

Alysia Zucker is studying for her bachelor of science with a major in Biology. She enjoys scuba diving, snowboarding, traveling, and working with children. She hopes to go to medical school so she can help people, just as the doctors helped her father.

Spin Zucker lives in Connecticut with his wife, Lori, and their daughter, Alysia. Spin is a peer counselor with NBMTLink, a national BMT support group. Spinzucker@aol.com.

Who Is
Jack Canfield?

J ack Canfield is the co-creator and editor of the Chicken Soup for the Soul series, which Time magazine has called "the publishing phenomenon of the decade." Jack is also the co-author of eight other bestselling books including *The Success Principles™: How to Get from Where You Are to Where You Want to Be*, *Dare to Win*, *The Aladdin Factor*, *You've Got to Read This Book*, and *The Power of Focus: How to Hit Your Business and Personal and Financial Targets with Absolute Certainty*.

Jack is the CEO of the Canfield Training Group in Santa Barbara, California, and founder of the Foundation for Self-Esteem in Culver City, California. He has conducted intensive personal and professional development seminars on the principles of success for over a million people in twenty-three countries. Jack is a dynamic keynote speaker and he has spoken to hundreds of thousands of others at more than 1,000 corporations, universities, professional conferences and conventions, and has been seen by millions more on national television shows such as *The Today Show*, *Fox and Friends*, *Inside Edition*, *Hard Copy*, CNN's *Talk Back Live*, *20/20*, *Eye to Eye*, and the *NBC Nightly News* and the *CBS Evening News*.

Jack is the recipient of many awards and honors, including three honorary doctorates and a Guinness World Records Certificate for having seven books from the *Chicken Soup for the Soul* series appearing on the New York Times bestseller list on May 24, 1998.

You can reach Jack at:

Jack Canfield
The Canfield Companies
P. O. Box 30880 • Santa Barbara, CA 93130
phone: 805-563-2935 • fax: 805-563-2945
www.jackcanfield.com

Mark Victor Hansen is the co-founder of Chicken Soup for the Soul, along with Jack Canfield. He is also a sought-after keynote speaker, bestselling author, and marketing maven. For more than thirty years, Mark's powerful messages of possibility, opportunity, and action have created powerful change in thousands of organizations and millions of individuals worldwide.

Mark's credentials include a lifetime of entrepreneurial success. He is a prolific writer with many bestselling books, such as *The One Minute Millionaire*, *Cracking the Millionaire Code*, *How to Make the Rest of Your Life the Best of Your Life*, *The Power of Focus*, *The Aladdin Factor*, and *Dare to Win*, in addition to the Chicken Soup for the Soul series. Mark has had a profound influence in the field of human potential through his library of audios, videos, and articles in the areas of big thinking, sales achievement, wealth building, publishing success, and personal and professional development. Mark is also the founder of the MEGA Seminar Series.

He has appeared on *Oprah*, CNN, and *The Today Show*. He has been quoted in *Time*, *U.S. News & World Report*, *USA Today*, *The New York Times*, and *Entrepreneur* and has given countless radio interviews, assuring our planet's people that "You can easily create the life you deserve."

Mark is the recipient of numerous awards that honor his entrepreneurial spirit, philanthropic heart, and business acumen. He is a lifetime member of the Horatio Alger Association of Distinguished Americans, an organization that honored Mark with the prestigious Horatio Alger Award for his extraordinary life achievements.

You can reach Mark at:

Mark Victor Hansen & Associates, Inc.
P. O. Box 7665 • Newport Beach, CA 92658
phone: 949-764-2640 • fax: 949-722-6912
www.markvictorhansen.com

Who Is
David Tabatsky?

David is a writer, editor, teacher, director and performing artist. He was the Consulting Editor for Marlo Thomas and her New York Times bestseller, *The Right Words at the Right Time, Volume 2: Your Turn* (Atria Books 2006).

David has published two editions of *What's Cool Berlin*, a comic travel guide to Germany's capital and written for *The Forward*, *Parenting* and *Sesame Street Parent*.

He has written and directed *A Whole Lotte Lenya*, a one-woman show inspired by the legendary actress and wife of Kurt Weill, which debuted at The Gene Frankel Theatre in New York, and *Standing in the Fuhrer's Slippers*, a work of historical fiction based on the life of Hitler's housekeeper, with touring scheduled for 2010.

David has worked professionally in theatre and circus as an actor, clown and juggler, appearing in New York at Lincoln Center, Radio City Music Hall, and the Beacon Theatre and throughout the United States, Europe, Russia and Japan, including his critically acclaimed solo performance at the Edinburgh Fringe Festival.

He played a significant role in the resurgence of the *Varieté* movement in Germany, with original shows at the *Chamaleon* in Berlin and the *Schmidt* in Hamburg, among others. He also directed *Kinderzirkus Taborka* at the renowned Tempodrom in Berlin.

David has taught and directed for the American School of London, die Etage in Berlin, the Big Apple Circus School, the United Nations International School and The Cathedral of St. John the Divine. He serves on the theatre faculty at Adelphi University and is a teaching artist for The Henry Street Settlement with a focus on special education.

He currently works with writers, developing memoirs, editing fiction and creating non-fiction projects of all kinds.

David lives in New York City with his children, Max and Stella. He can be reached through his website: www.tabatsky.com.

Acknowledgments

Thanks to Amy Newmark, a great publisher and editor.

Thanks to D'ette Corona, Barbara LoMonaco, and Kristiana Glavin for their administrative support and editorial skills.

Thanks to Brian Taylor, our book designer, for superior execution of this unique book-within-a-book project.

Thanks to Nelsie Spencer and Bruce Kluger for their moral support.

Thanks to Lauren Singer Katz for her excellent and cheerful assistance.

Thanks to all of the contributing authors and their families.

Thanks to all those who submitted stories we weren't able to accept. We read every one, and even those that were not used helped to shape this book.

Thanks to Max and Stella.

And to Irene Tabatsky, whose memory has graced these pages.

Resources Mentioned in the Stories

American Cancer Society's Relay For Life
Relay For Life brings together more than 3.5 million people to celebrate the lives of those who have battled cancer.
www.acs.org

American Society of Clinical Oncology
Professional organization for physicians who treat cancer.
www.asco.org

Camp Goodtimes
Established in 1985 by the Canadian Cancer Society and serving children, as well as their families, with a history of cancer.
www.cancer.ca or gotcamp@bc.cancer.ca

The CancerClimber Association (CCA)
Our mission is to help those touched by cancer by focusing on living an active, healthy lifestyle.
www.keep-climbing.org

CaringBridge
Free, personalized websites, connect loved ones during critical illness, treatment and recovery.
www.caringbridge.org

Clown Care
The Big Apple Circus's signature community outreach program brings the joy of the classical circus to hospitalized children at 19 leading pediatric facilities across the United States.
www.bigapplecircus.org/community/clown-care

Dana-Farber Cancer Institute
An independent institution of over 4,000 staff members, the teaching affiliate of Harvard Medical School specializes in cancer research and pediatric and adult patient care.
www.dana-farber.org

Hole in the Wall Gang camps
Paul Newman founded the first in what has grown to become the world's largest family of camps serving children with serious illnesses.
www.holeinthewallgang.org

I'm Too Young For This!
An advocacy, support and research organization, working exclusively on behalf of survivors and care providers under the age of forty.
www.imtooyoungforthis.org

Johns Hopkins Avon Foundation Breast Center
A comprehensive breast care program, offering a full spectrum of clinical and support services, from screening and diagnosis to treatment and counseling.
www.hopkinsbreastcenter.org

Lotsa Helping Hands
A simple way for friends, family, colleagues, and neighbors to assist loved ones in need, designed for organizing help during times of medical crisis.
www.lotsahelpinghands.com

Melissa's Living Legacy Foundation
Resources to help teens with cancer meet their life challenges in productive and satisfying ways.
www.teenslivingwithcancer.org

Roswell Park Cancer Institute
A comprehensive cancer center (research and treatment) located in Buffalo, New York.
www.roswellpark.org

Sunrise Day Camp
The only dedicated day camp in the nation for children with cancer, situated on Long Island, New York. Offered free of charge on a non-sectarian basis.
www.sunrisedaycamp.org

Susan G. Komen Race for the Cure
The world's largest grassroots network of breast cancer survivors and activists fighting to save lives and ensure quality care for all and energize science to find the cures.
www.komen.org

St. Jude Children's Research Hospital
With research and patent care under one roof, St. Jude makes revolutionary discoveries happen. All patients accepted are treated without regard to the family's ability to pay.
www.stjude.org

The Lydia Project
A network of support and prayerful encouragement for women in Augusta, nationwide, and beyond. Women are typically welcomed with a beautiful tote made with love by volunteers.
www.thelydiaproject.org

Wayland Angels
A volunteer group, which began serving families in crisis in 2003.
www.waylandangels.org

Chicken Soup for the Soul

Improving Your Life Every Day

Real people sharing real stories—for fifteen years. Now, Chicken Soup for the Soul has gone beyond the bookstore to become a world leader in life improvement. Through books, movies, DVDs, online resources and other partnerships, we bring hope, courage, inspiration and love to hundreds of millions of people around the world. Chicken Soup for the Soul's writers and readers belong to a one-of-a-kind global community, sharing advice, support, guidance, comfort, and knowledge.

Chicken Soup for the Soul stories have been translated into more than forty languages and can be found in more than one hundred countries. Every day, millions of people experience a Chicken Soup for the Soul story in a book, magazine, newspaper or online. As we share our life experiences through these stories, we offer hope, comfort and inspiration to one another. The stories travel from person to person, and from country to country, helping to improve lives everywhere.

Share with Us

We all have had Chicken Soup for the Soul moments in our lives. If you would like to share your story or poem with millions of people around the world, go to www.chickensoup.com and click on "Submit Your Story." You may be able to help another reader, and become a published author at the same time. Some of our past contributors have launched writing and speaking careers from the publication of their stories in our books!

Your stories have the best chance of being used if you submit them through our website, at

www.chickensoup.com

If you do not have access to the Internet, you may submit your stories by mail or by facsimile. Please do not send us any book manuscripts, unless through a literary agent, as these will be automatically discarded.

Chicken Soup for the Soul
P.O. Box 700
Cos Cob, CT 06807-0700
Fax 203-861-7194